BBC goodfood
5 INGREDIENTS

D1341391

BBC goodfood

5 INGREDIENTS

130 SIMPLE DISHES FOR EVERY DAY OF THE WEEK

BBC BOOKS

10 9 8 7 6 5 4 3 2 1

BBC Books, an imprint of Ebury Publishing
20 Vauxhall Bridge Road,
London SW1V 2SA

BBC Books is part of the Penguin Random House
group of companies whose addresses can be
found at global.penguinrandomhouse.com

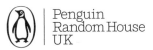

Photographs © BBC Magazines 2018
Recipes © BBC Worldwide 2018
Book design © Woodlands Books Ltd 2018
All recipes contained in this book first appeared in
BBC *Good Food* magazine.

First published by BBC Books in 2018

www.eburypublishing.co.uk

A CIP catalogue record for this book is available
from the British Library

ISBN 9781785943935

Colour origination by BORN Ltd
Typeset in India by Integra Software Services
Pvt. Ltd
Printed and bound in China by C&C Offset Printing
Co, Ltd.

Cover Design: Interstate Creative Partners Ltd
Production: Rebecca Jones

Penguin Random House is committed to a
sustainable future for our business, our readers and
our planet. This book is made from Forest
Stewardship Council® certified paper.

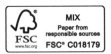

BBC Books would like to thank the following people
for providing photos. While every effort has been
made to trace and acknowledge all photographers,
we should like to apologise should there be any
errors or omissions.

Image credits:
Emma Boyns 275, 277; Peter Cassidy 49, 107, 177, 195,
197; Mike English 13, 17, 31, 39, 43, 47, 63, 77, 93, 127,
129, 133, 141, 155, 157, 161, 169, 175, 179, 181, 183, 185,
187, 189, 193, 201, 211, 213, 219, 231, 235, 281; Will
Heap 19, 21, 115, 119, 165, 173, 237, 255, 257, 259, 261,
263, 269, 283; Adrian Lawrence 225; Gareth
Morgans 27, 121, 223, 271; David Munns 41, 57, 65, 69,
105, 147, 153, 239, 245; Myles New 33, 55, 229; Stuart
Ovenden 6, 8, 25, 61, 67, 75, 103, 139, 149, 167, 171,
191, 205, 209, 217, 253; Lis Parsons 221; Tom Regester
29, 37, 101, 117, 125, 131, 135, 137, 143, 145, 163, 203,
215, 233, 243, 265, 273; Craig Robertson 85; Toby
Scott 15; Maja Smend 95; Sam Stowell 81, 83, 87, 89,
91, 97, 99, 109, 207, 249; Rob Streeter 51, 247;
unknown 73, 111, 227, 267; Simon Walton 151; Philip
Webb 71, 251; Jon Whitaker 45, 279; Clare Winfield
23, 35, 59, 123.

All the recipes in this book were created by the
editorial team at Good Food and by regular
contributors to BBC Magazines.

Contents

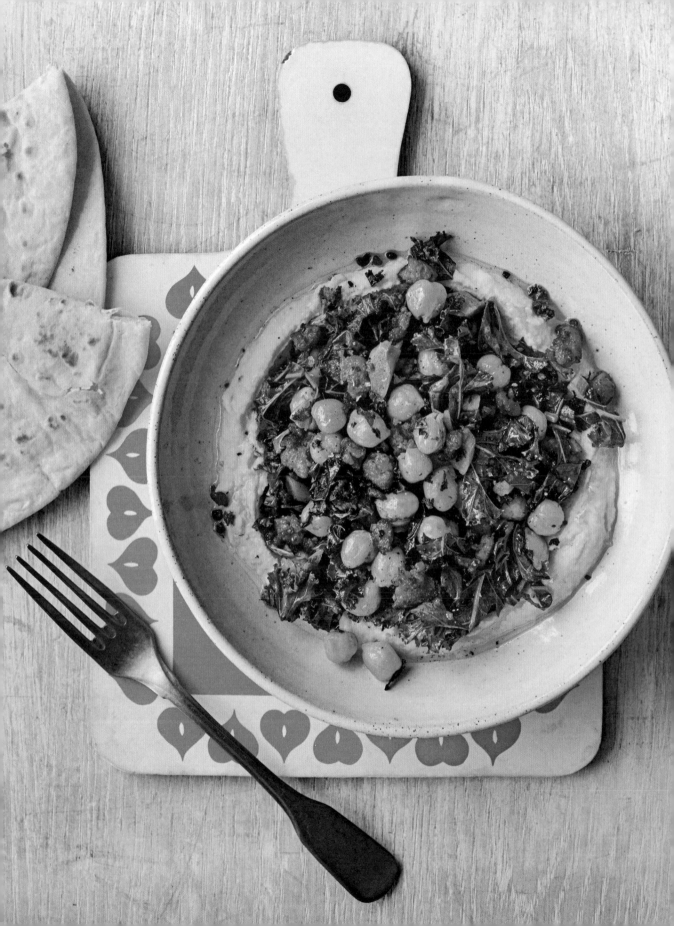

Introduction

Busy lives and the convenience of ready meals and takeaways can mean less time in the kitchen for many of us, but it doesn't have to be that way. This book is full of quick and simple recipes, all of which use 5 ingredients or less (excluding a few store cupboard staples) guaranteed to get you cooking more.

The benefits of cooking with so few ingredients are threefold: A quick dash around the shops on your way home and you're ready to cook (you'll probably already have a few ingredients in the cupboards). Less ingredients equals less time chopping and preparing, and so lots of the recipes in this book are quick to prepare. Finally, these recipes are all easy to remember, for those days when you're in need of some inspiration all you need to do is remember a handful of ingredients and, hey presto, you can whip up something delicious in no time at all.

This handy book isn't all about dinner. It has new ideas for breakfasts, starters, sides and desserts too. Five ingredients means ease, so if you want simple cooking for all occasions we've got it covered. Smoothies, pancakes and loaded bagels are all on the menu for breakfast and you won't believe the desserts you can make with just 5 ingredients – Chocolate hazelnut cheesecake anyone? Or how about warm cinnamon buns?

One thing you never have to worry about when cooking a *Good Food* recipe is if the recipe will work. We triple test all of our recipes in our development kitchen, tweaking and adapting until it's just right, meaning all you have to do is follow the recipe for perfect results. The recipes in this book are all nutritionally analysed by a qualified nutritionist so you can see at a glance how they will impact your diet. We pride ourselves in offering recipes for every cook, meaning we choose ingredients that are easy to get hold of in most supermarkets, or if it's something special, online.

With this book in your kitchen everyday cooking can become such a joy. Long ingredient lists are a thing of the past, and are not always necessary for turning out great food. There's something for every occasion, and recipes you'll turn to time and time again. These trustworthy, easy recipes will be loved by the whole family, so get cooking!

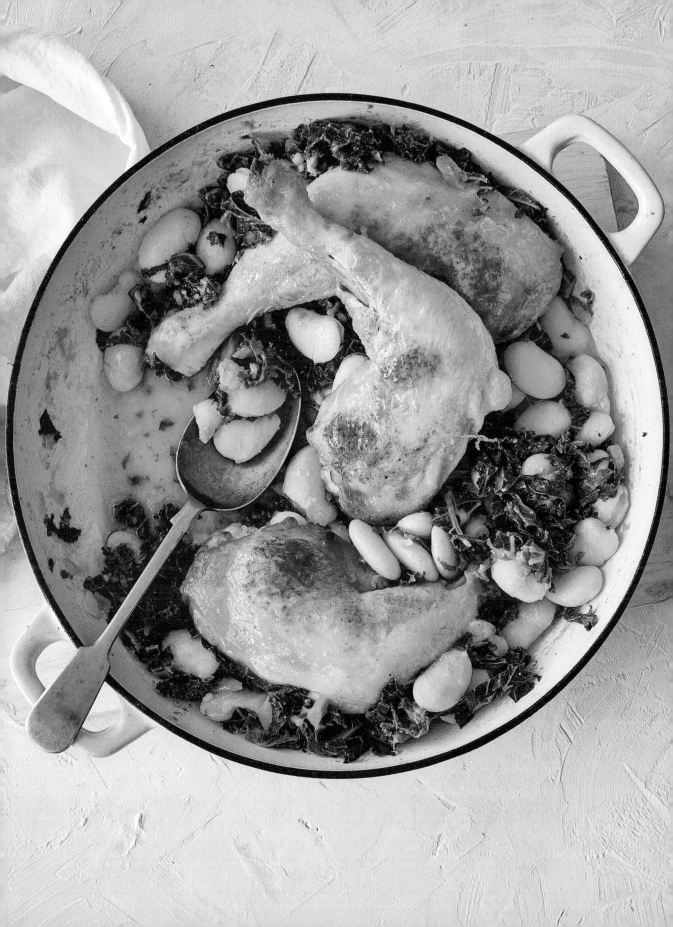

Notes & conversions

STORE CUPBOARD

Most people will have oil, salt and pepper in their cupboards, so we haven't counted these as one of the five ingredients in the recipes. However, we have left them in the ingredients lists to make the recipes easier for you to follow.

NOTES ON THE RECIPES

- Eggs are large in the UK and Australia and extra large in America unless stated.
- Wash fresh produce before preparation.
- Recipes contain nutritional analyses for 'sugars', which means the total sugar content including all natural sugars in the ingredients, unless otherwise stated.

APPROXIMATE LIQUID CONVERSION

Metric	Imperial	Aus	US
50ml	2 fl oz	¼ cup	¼ cup
125ml	4 fl oz	½ cup	½ cup
175ml	6 fl oz	¾ cup	¾ cup
225ml	8 fl oz	1 cup	1 cup
300ml	10 fl oz/½ pint	½ pint	1¼ cups
450ml	16 fl oz	2 cups	2 cups/1 pint
600ml	20 fl oz/1 pint	1 pint	2½ cups
1 litre	35 fl oz/1¾ pints	1¾ pints	1 quart

OVEN TEMPERATURE CONVERSION

GAS	°C	°C FAN	°F	OVEN TEMP.
¼	110	90	225	Very cool
½	120	100	250	Very cool
1	140	120	275	Cool or slow
2	150	130	300	Cool or slow
3	160	140	325	Warm
4	180	160	350	Moderate
5	190	170	375	Moderately hot
6	200	180	400	Fairly hot
7	220	200	425	Hot
8	230	210	450	Very hot
9	240	220	475	Very hot

APPROXIMATE WEIGHT CONVERSIONS

Cup measurements, which are used in Australia and America, have not been listed here as they vary from ingredient to ingredient. Kitchen scales should be used to measure dry/solid ingredients.

SPOON MEASURES

Spoon measurements are level unless otherwise specifed.

- 1 teaspoon (tsp) = 5ml
- 1 tablespoon (tbsp) = 15ml
- 1 Australian tablespoon = 20ml (cooks in Australia should measure 3 teaspoons where 1 tablespoon is specifed in a recipe)

Good Food is concerned about sustainable sourcing and animal welfare. Where possible, humanely reared meats, sustainably caught fish (see fishonline.org for further information from the Marine Conservation Society) and free-range chickens and eggs are used when recipes are originally tested.

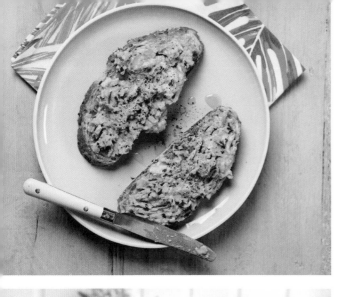

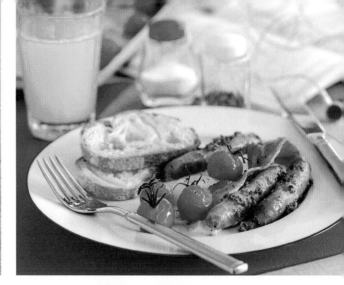

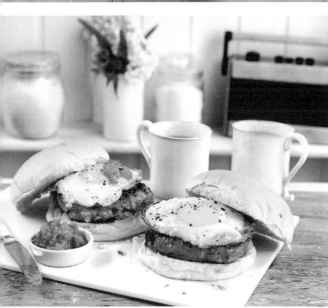

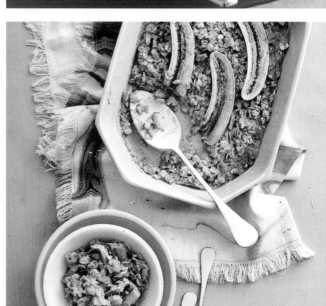

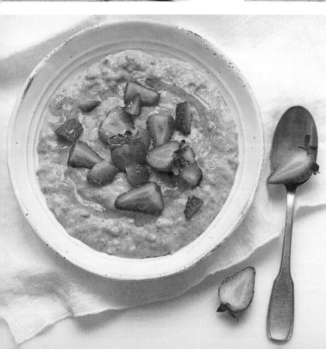

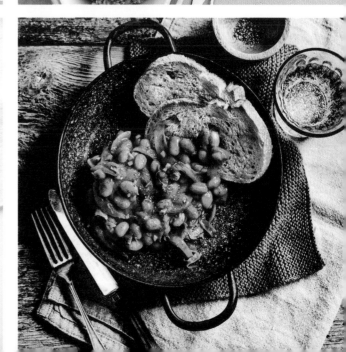

CHAPTER 1: BREAKFASTS & BRUNCHES

Want a quick, simple breakfast but getting bored of the same old cereal and toast? This chapter is packed with exciting new ideas to make breakfast worth waking up for. We've got a one-pan Smoky shakshuka, a smoothie bowl, frittata and even a big fry-up for the weekend, all in 5 ingredients or less, giving you more time to kick back, read the papers and enjoy your mornings.

Smoky shakshuka

Our easy version of the North African dish contains chorizo, roasted red peppers, tomatoes and eggs – eat it for breakfast, lunch or dinner!

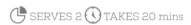 SERVES 2 TAKES 20 mins

- ½ a ring of chorizo
- 2 roasted red peppers, from a jar
- 400g can chopped tomatoes
- 2 eggs
- toast, to serve

1 Slice the chorizo and cook in a frying pan until the oils are released. Slice the peppers, add to the pan with the tomatoes, season and cook until warmed through.

2 Make 2 spaces in the pan and crack an egg into each one. Cover with a lid and simmer for 5 mins until the eggs are cooked. Serve with toast.

Nutrition per serving
Kcals 348 • fat 23g • saturates 8g • carbs 11g • sugars 8g • fibre 2g • protein 23g • salt 2.2g

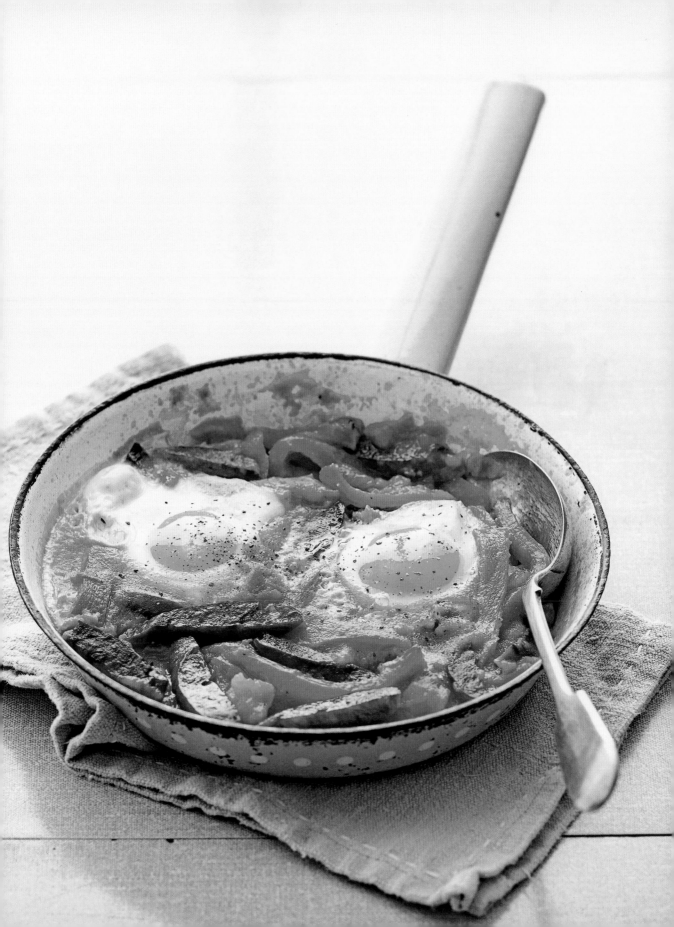

Baked green eggs

This 5-ingredient breakfast or brunch with spinach, pesto and bubbling melted cheese can be on the table in 15 minutes.

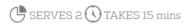 SERVES 2 ⏱ TAKES 15 mins

- 100g baby spinach, roughly chopped
- 4 tbsp fresh pesto
- 100ml double cream
- 1 tbsp finely grated Gruyère (or vegetarian alternative)
- 4 medium eggs

1 Heat oven to 200C/180C fan/gas 6. Mix together the spinach, pesto, cream and some seasoning, and tip into 2 individual shallow ovenproof dishes. Sprinkle the cheese over the top. Make 2 shallow hollows in the mixture in each dish and break an egg into each hollow. Bake in the oven for 10–12 mins until the whites are set and the yolks are still runny.

Nutrition per serving
Kcals 579 • fat 54g • saturates 23g • carbs 3g • sugars 3g • fibre 3g • protein 19g • salt 1.5g

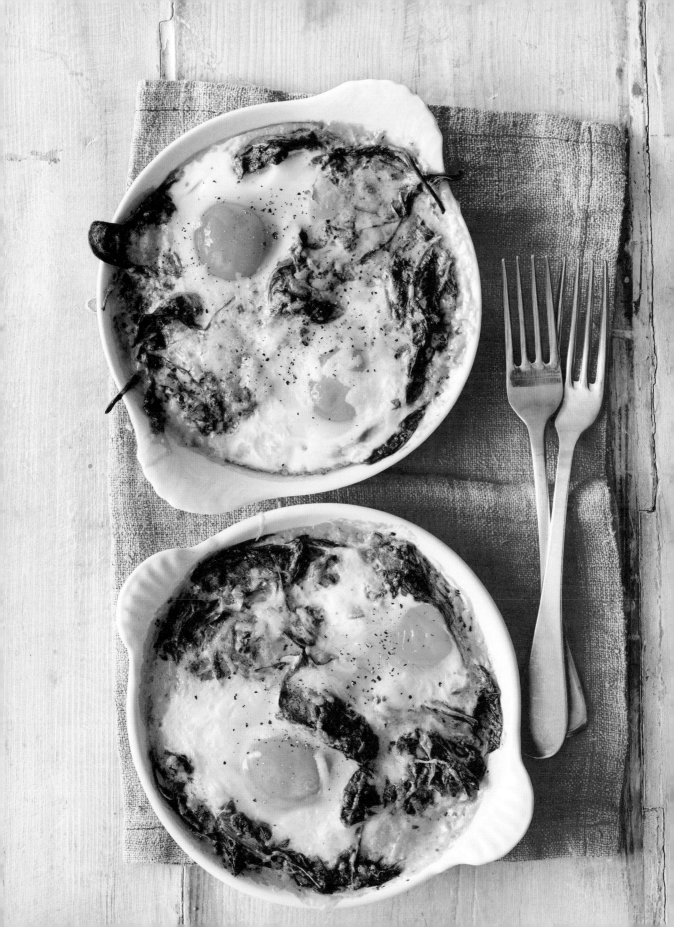

Asparagus & new potato frittata

A simple, low-calorie spring main that uses the season's finest ingredients and is ready in just 20 minutes.

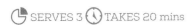 SERVES 3 TAKES 20 mins

- 200g new potatoes, quartered
- 100g asparagus tips
- 1 tbsp olive oil
- 1 onion, finely chopped
- 6 eggs, beaten
- 40g cheddar, grated

1 Heat the grill to high. Put the potatoes in a pan of cold salted water and bring to the boil. Once boiling, cook for 4–5 mins until nearly tender, then add the asparagus for a final 1 min. Drain.

2 Meanwhile, heat the oil in an ovenproof frying pan and add the onion. Cook for about 8 mins until softened.

3 Mix the eggs with half the cheese in a jug and season well. Pour over the onion in the pan, then scatter over the asparagus and potatoes. Top with the remaining cheese and put under the grill for 5 mins or until golden and cooked through. Cut into wedges and serve from the pan with salad.

Nutrition per serving
Kcals 310 • fat 18g • saturates 6g • carbs 16g • sugars 6g • fibre 4g • protein 19g • salt 0.7g

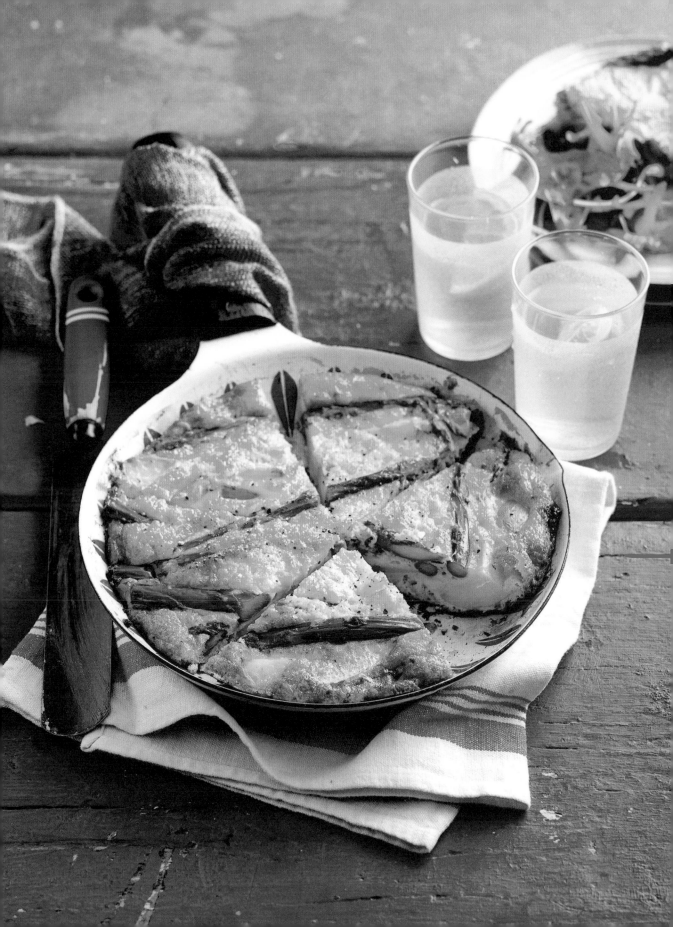

Avocado on toast

Make this simple speedy breakfast with just a handful of ingredients. Our avocado toast uses crusty sourdough bread and a pinch of chilli for a kick.

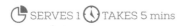 SERVES 1 TAKES 5 mins

- 1 ripe avocado
- ½ lemon
- big pinch chilli flakes
- 2 slices sourdough bread
- good drizzle extra virgin olive oil

1 Cut the avocado in half and carefully remove its stone, then scoop out the flesh into a bowl. Squeeze in the lemon juice then mash with a fork to your desired texture. Season to taste with sea salt, black pepper and chilli flakes. Toast your bread, drizzle over the olive oil, then pile the avocado on top.

Nutrition per serving
Kcals 501 • fat 33g • saturates 7g • carbs 37g • sugars 3g • fibre 9g • protein 10g • salt 1.2g

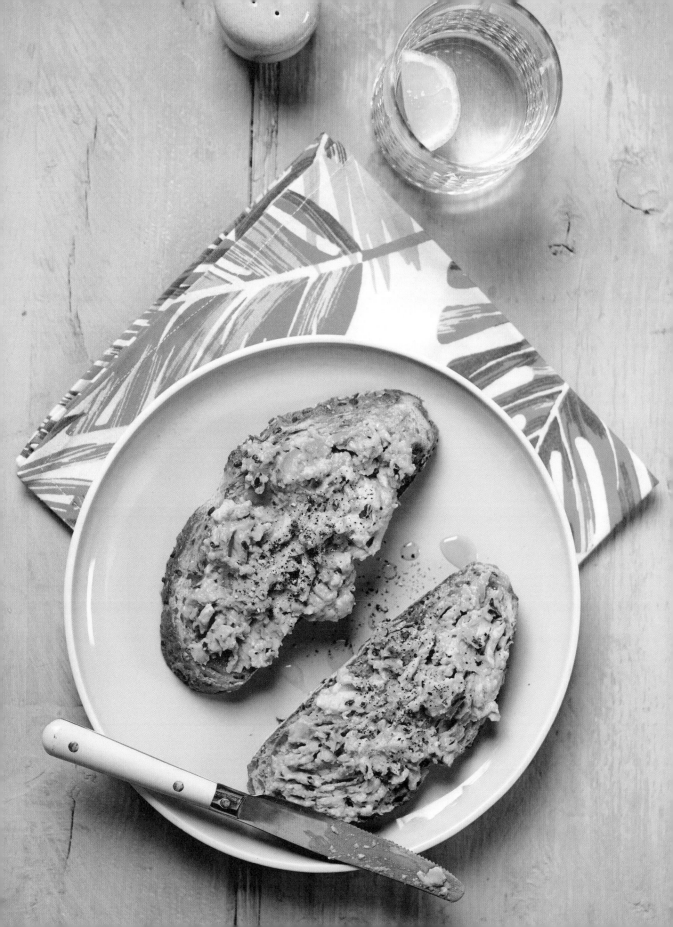

Hash browns

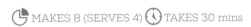

Crispy hash browns are a must for the full English breakfast. With just 3 ingredients and being freezeable, too, they're easy to add to your next fry up.

 MAKES 8 (SERVES 4) TAKES 30 mins

- 3 medium potatoes (approx. 370g in total, unpeeled, left whole – Maris Pipers, King Edward and Desirée are good choices)
- 50g butter, melted
- 4 tbsp sunflower oil

1 Cook the potatoes in a saucepan of boiling water for 10 mins, then drain and set aside until they are cool enough to handle.

2 Coarsely grate the potatoes into a bowl discarding any skin that comes off in your hand as you grate. Season well with salt and pepper and pour over half the butter. Mix well then divide the mix into 8 and shape into patties or squares. The hash browns can be prepared a day ahead and chilled until ready to cook or frozen for up to a month.

3 To cook, heat the oil and the remaining butter in a frying pan until sizzling and gently fry the hash browns, in batches if needed, for 4–5 mins on each side until crisp and golden. Serve straight away or leave in a low oven to keep warm.

Nutrition per serving
Kcals 264 • fat 21g • saturates 8g • carbs 16g • sugars 1g • fibre 2g • protein 2g • salt 0.4g

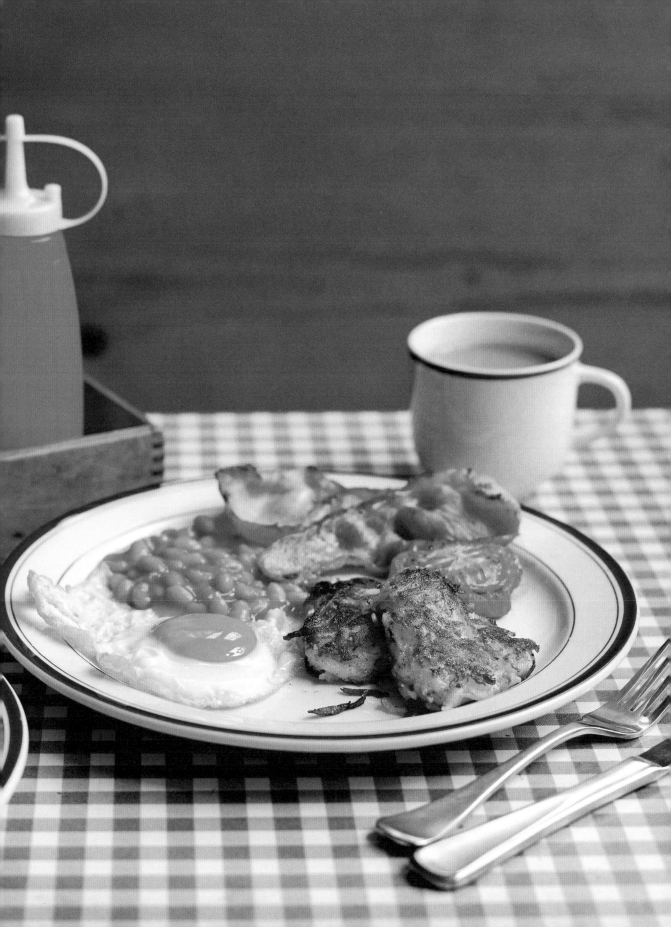

Banana pancakes

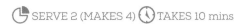

Gluten-free banana pancakes you can whip up in just 10 minutes! Scatter with pecans and raspberries to enjoy a low-calorie yet indulgent breakfast.

SERVE 2 (MAKES 4) TAKES 10 mins

- 1 large banana
- 2 medium eggs, beaten
- pinch of baking powder (gluten-free if coeliac)
- 1 tsp oil
- 25g pecans, roughly chopped
- 125g raspberries

1 In a bowl, mash the banana with a fork until it resembles a thick purée. Stir in the egg and baking powder.
2 Heat a large non-stick frying pan or pancake pan over a medium heat and brush with half the oil. Using half the batter, spoon 2 pancakes into the pan, cook for 1–2 mins each side, then tip onto a plate. Repeat the process with the remaining oil and batter. Top the pancakes with the pecans and raspberries.

Nutrition per serving
Kcals 243 • fat 15g • saturates 2g • carbs 15g • sugars 14g • fibre 4g • protein 9g • salt 0.3g

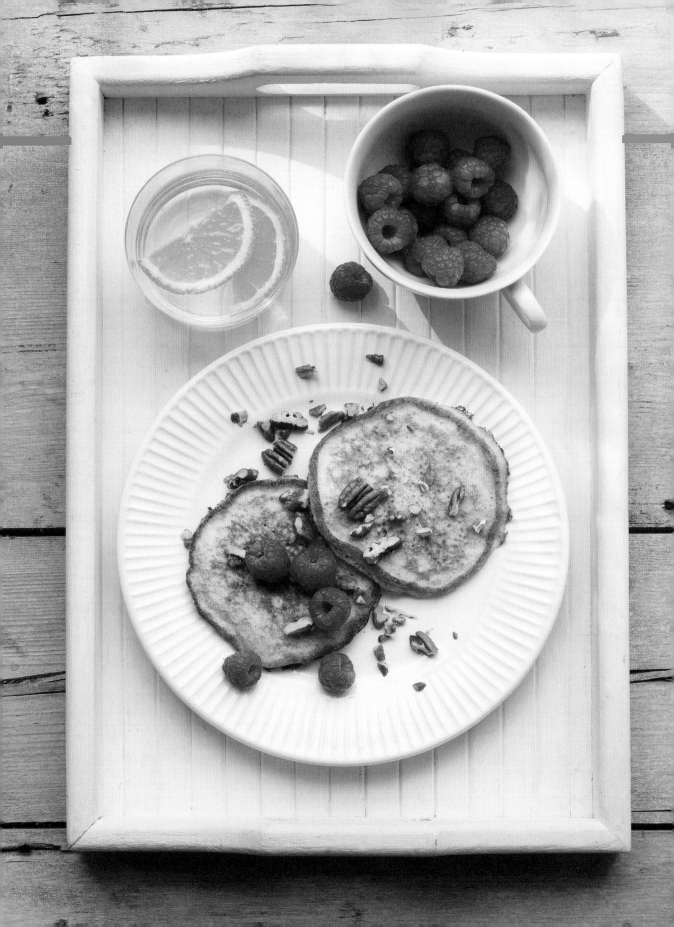

Veggie breakfast bakes

Hit three of your 5-a-day with this alternative fry-up – it's packed with vegetables and oven-baked.

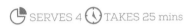 SERVES 4 TAKES 25 mins

- 4 large field mushrooms
- 8 tomatoes, halved
- 1 garlic clove, thinly sliced
- 2 tsp olive oil
- 200g bag spinach
- 4 eggs

1 Heat oven to 200C/180C fan/gas 6. Put the mushrooms and tomatoes into 4 ovenproof dishes. Divide the garlic among the dishes, drizzle over the oil and some seasoning, then bake for 10 mins.

2 Meanwhile, put the spinach into a large colander, then pour over a kettle of boiling water to wilt it. Squeeze out any excess water, then add the spinach to the dishes. Make a little gap between the vegetables and crack an egg into each dish. Return the dishes to the oven and cook for a further 8–10 mins or until the egg is cooked to your liking.

Nutrition per serving
Kcals 127 • fat 8g • saturates 2g • carbs 5g • sugars 5g • fibre 3g • protein 9g • salt 0.4g

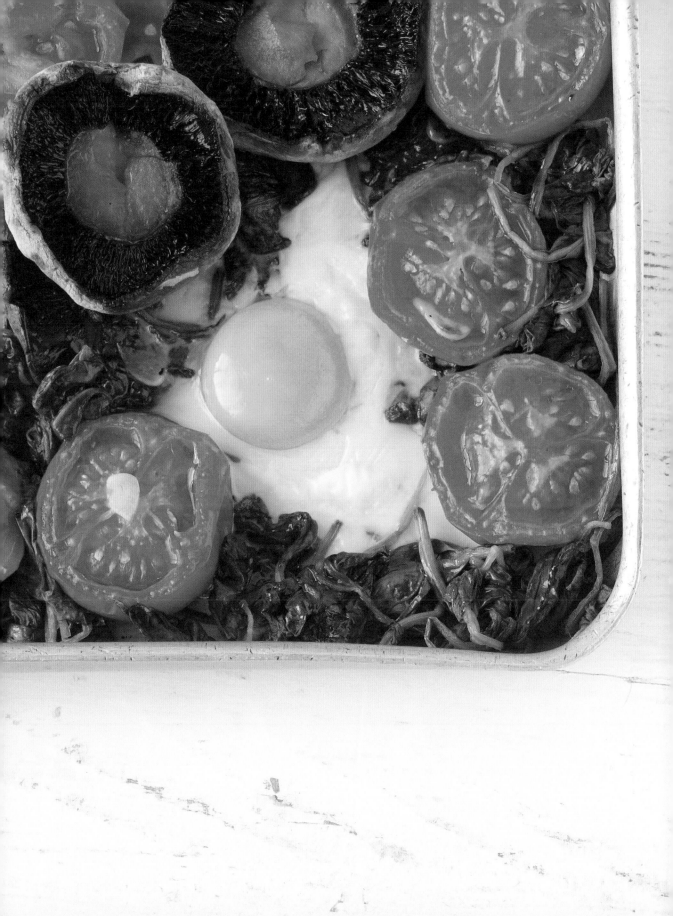

All-day breakfast

If you've woken up with a sore head and can't face juggling pans for a fry-up, try this one-tray breakfast.

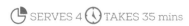 SERVES 4 🕐 TAKES 35 mins

- 1 pack chipolata sausages
- 1 tbsp olive oil
- 8 bacon rashers
- small punnet cherry tomatoes, about 250g
- 2 tsp wholegrain mustard
- 4 eggs

1 Heat oven to 220C/200C fan/gas 7. Toss the sausages and oil in a shallow roasting tin, then spread out in an even layer. Drape bacon rashers over the top and roast for 15–20 mins until both are starting to brown and sizzle.

2 Move the bacon and sausages around so everything browns evenly. Scatter over the tomatoes and blob the mustard onto the sausages. Use a pair of tongs or a spoon to create 4 gaps for the eggs, then crack an egg into each gap. Put the tin back in the oven for 5–8 mins or until the egg whites are set and tomatoes softening.

Nutrition per serving
Kcals 587 • fat 48g • saturates 15g • carbs 13g • sugars 5g • fibre 2g • protein 28g • salt 3.67g

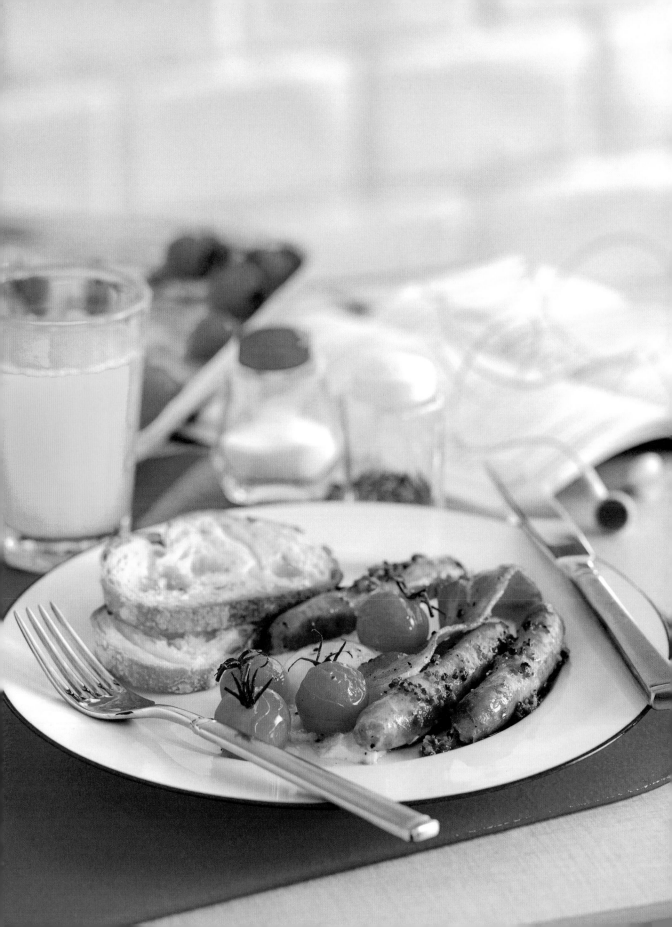

Mushroom brunch

You only need mushrooms, eggs, kale and garlic to cook this tasty one-pan brunch. It's comforting yet healthy, low-calorie and gluten-free too …

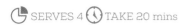 SERVES 4 TAKE 20 mins

- 250g mushrooms
- 1 garlic clove
- 1 tbsp olive oil
- 160g bag kale
- 4 eggs

1 Slice the mushrooms and crush the garlic clove. Heat the olive oil in a large non-stick frying pan, then fry the garlic over a low heat for 1 min. Add the mushrooms and cook until soft, then add the kale. If the kale won't all fit in the pan, add half and stir until wilted, then add the rest. Once all the kale is wilted, season.

2 Now crack in the eggs and keep them cooking gently for 2–3 mins. Cover with the lid for a further 2–3 mins or until the eggs are cooked to your liking. Serve with bread.

Nutrition per serving
Kcals 154 • fat 11g • saturates 2g • carbs 1g • sugars 1g • fibre 2g • protein 13g • salt 0.4g

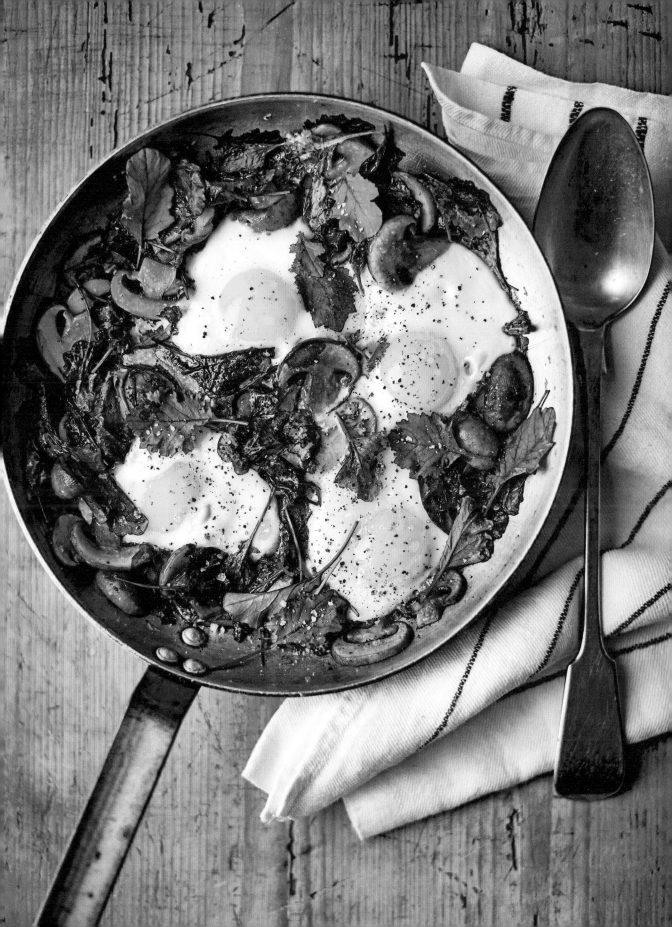

Baked banana porridge

Start the day right with this healthy baked banana porridge containing walnuts, banana and cinnamon. It's a filling breakfast that will keep you going until lunch.

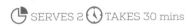 SERVES 2 TAKES 30 mins

- 2 small bananas, halved lengthways
- 100g jumbo porridge oats
- ¼ tsp cinnamon
- 150ml milk of your choice, plus extra to serve
- 4 walnuts, roughly chopped

1 Heat oven to 190C/170C fan/gas 5. Mash up 1 banana half, then mix it with the oats, cinnamon, milk, 300ml water and a pinch of salt, and pour into a baking dish. Top with the remaining banana halves and scatter over the walnuts.

2 Bake for 20–25 mins until the oats are creamy and have absorbed most of the liquid.

Nutrition per serving
Kcals 405 • fat 15g • saturates 2g • carbs 52g • sugars 18g • fibre 6g • protein 12g • salt 0.3g

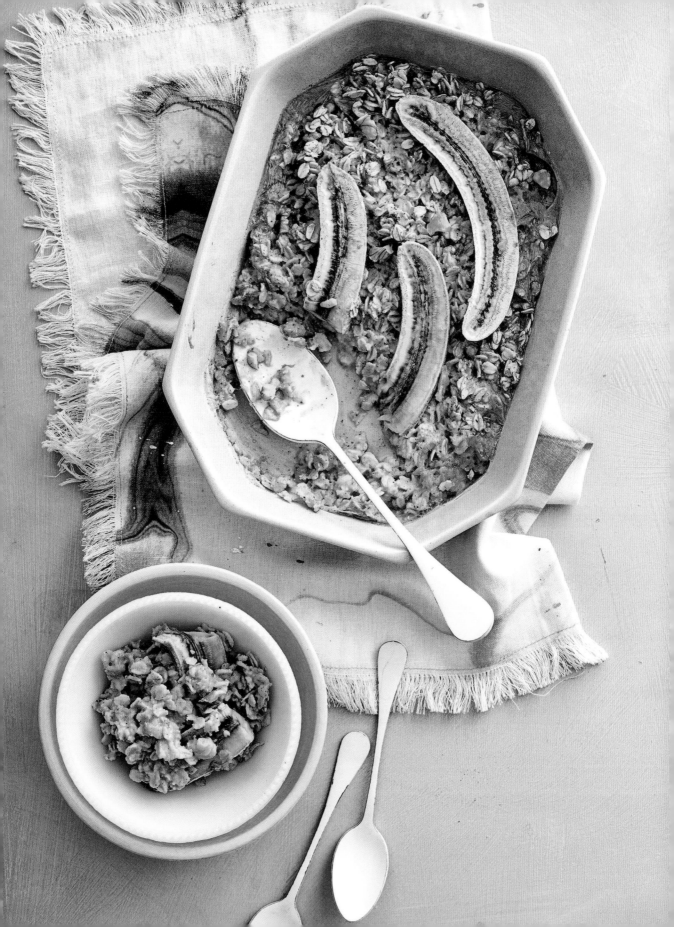

Blueberry bircher pots

Avoid the lure of the muffin and latte. These snacks help beat off the mid-morning munchies.

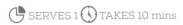 SERVES 1 TAKES 10 mins

- 1 small apple
- 2 tbsp porridge oats
- 2 tbsp low-fat natural yogurt
- pinch of cinnamon
- small handful blueberries

1 Grate the apple and mix with the oats, yogurt and cinnamon. Layer in a pot with the blueberries.

Nutrition per pot
Kcals 222 • fat 3g • saturates 0.7g • carbs 38g • sugars 20g • fibre 7g • protein 8g • salt 0.1g

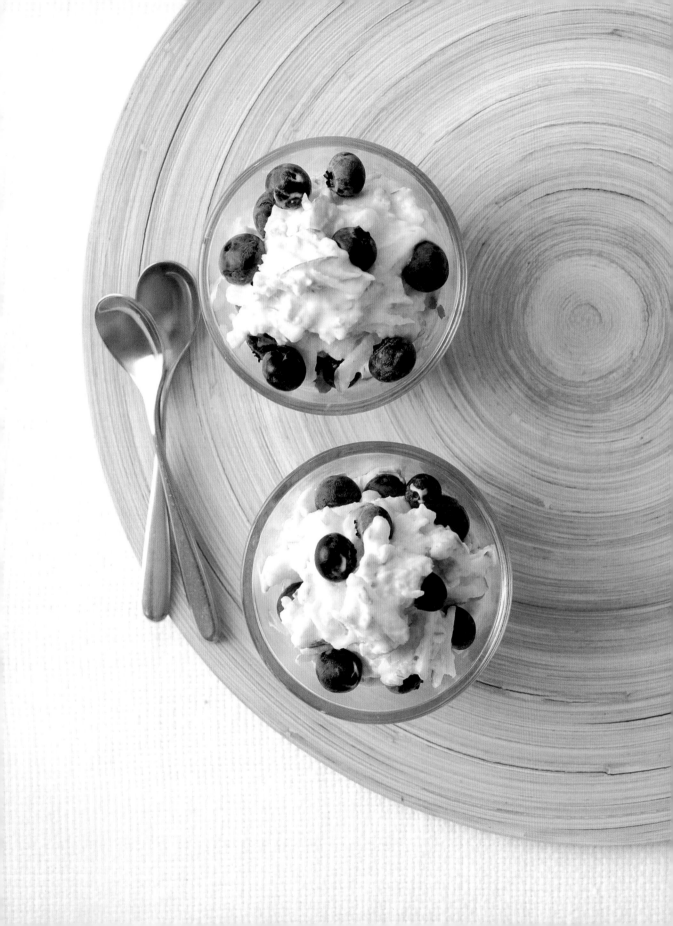

Three grain porridge

This healthy breakfast, made from toasted oatmeal, spelt and barley, is super simple to make and can be kept for up to 6 months.

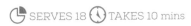 SERVES 18 TAKES 10 mins

- 300g oatmeal
- 300g spelt flakes
- 300g barley flakes
- agave nectar and sliced strawberries, to serve (optional)

1 Working in batches, toast the oatmeal, spelt flakes and barley in a large, dry frying pan for 5 mins until golden, then leave to cool and store in an airtight container.

2 When you want to eat it, simply combine 50g of the porridge mixture in a saucepan with 300ml milk or water. Cook for 5 mins, stirring occasionally, then top with a drizzle of agave nectar and strawberries, if you like (optional). Will keep for 6 months.

Nutrition per serving
Kcals 179 • fat 2g • saturates 0g • carbs 32g • sugars 1g • fibre 4g • protein 7g • salt 0g

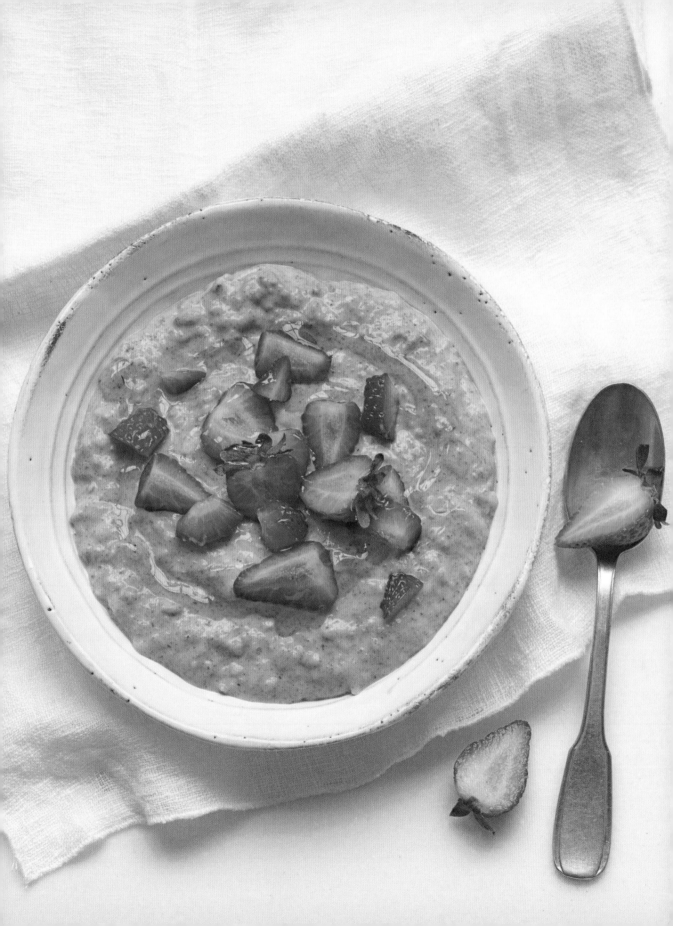

Matcha breakfast bowl

Mix nutritious matcha powder with natural yogurt in this maple syrup and fruit-topped breakfast that's 2 of your 5-a-day ...

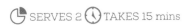 SERVES 2 ⏱ TAKES 15 mins

- 300g natural yogurt
- 1 tbsp matcha powder
- 2 tsp maple syrup
- fresh fruit, to serve
- 20g coconut flakes, toasted

1 Mix the yogurt with the matcha and maple syrup, and divide between 2 bowls. Top with the fruit. Sprinkle over the coconut flakes just before serving.

Nutrition per serving
Kcals 261 • fat 11g • saturates 8g • carbs 27g • sugars 26g • fibre 5g • protein 10g • salt 0.3g

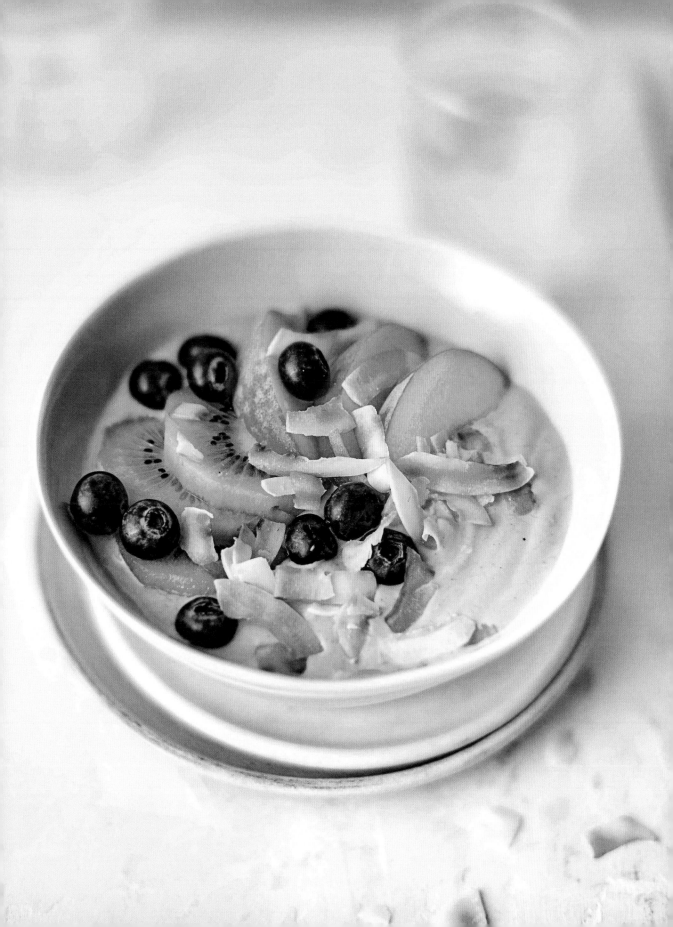

Breakfast beans

Enjoy this slow-cooked alternative to canned baked beans for breakfast or brunch, served on toast or with eggs. They're a good source of protein.

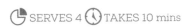 SERVES 4 ⏱ TAKES 10 mins

- 1 tbsp olive oil
- 1 onion, thinly sliced
- 1 tbsp white or red wine vinegar
- 400g can pinto beans, drained and rinsed
- 200ml passata
- small bunch coriander, chopped

1 Heat the oil in a large frying pan and fry the onion until it starts to brown. Add the vinegar and bubble for a minute. Stir in the beans and passata and season with black pepper.
2 Cook for 5 mins, until the sauce thickens and the beans are hot. Stir through the coriander.

Nutrition per serving
Kcals 149 • fat 3g • saturates 0.5g • carbs 21g • sugars 12g • fibre 5g • protein 6g • salt 0.39g

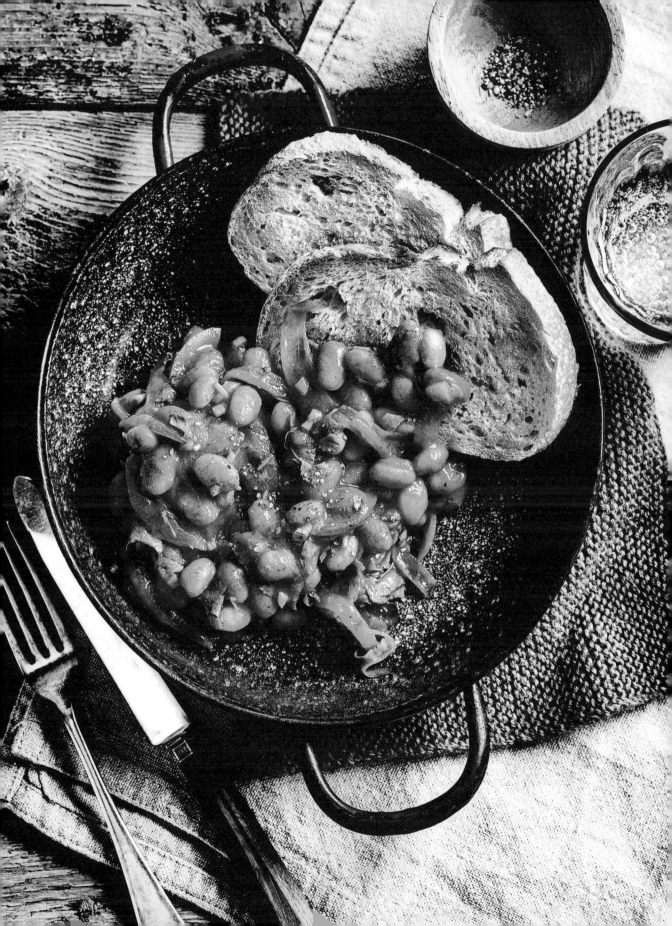

Big breakfast with asparagus

Cut down on the washing up by cooking everything in the oven with this no-fuss 'fry-up' of bacon, black pudding and eggs.

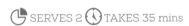 SERVES 2 TAKES 35 mins

- 6 rashers streaky dry-cured bacon
- 2 fat slices black pudding
- 12 asparagus spears (after snapping off woody ends)
- 1 tsp sunflower oil
- 2 eggs

1 Heat oven to 220C/200C fan/gas 7. Arrange the bacon and black pudding in a shallow roasting tin that's large enough for all the ingredients to fit snugly. Roast for 10 mins until the bacon is starting to crisp up, then turn over the bacon and black pudding and cook for another 5 mins.

2 Toss the asparagus in the oil and season, then add to the tin in bunches. Roast for another 5 mins, then remove from the oven and turn the asparagus, leaving 2 holes for the eggs. Crack an egg into each gap and put back in the oven for 4–5 mins until the whites are just set but the yolks are still runny. Serve immediately, straight from the tin, with toast and your choice of sauce.

Nutrition per serving
Kcals 534 • fat 39g • saturates 14g • carbs 14g • sugars 2g • fibre 2g • protein 30g • salt 4.8g

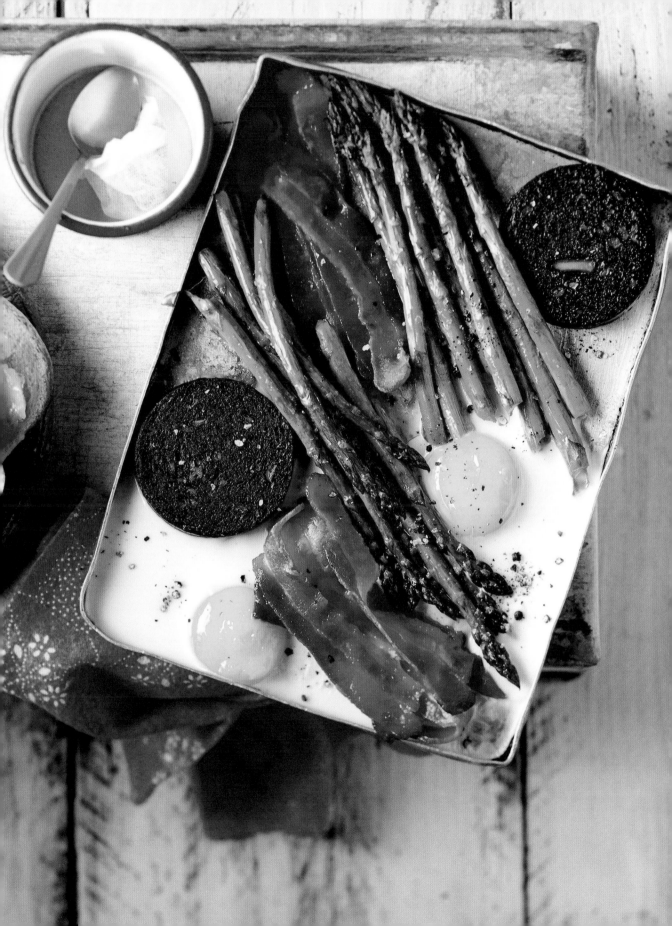

Breakfast bagel club

Salty, smoky and creamy, this made-in-minutes toasted bagel with cream cheese, smoked salmon and avocado is ideal for Sunday brunch.

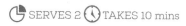 SERVES 2 ⏲ TAKES 10 mins

- 50g cream cheese
- 2 bagels, halved and lightly toasted
- 100g smoked salmon, cut into slices
- 1 avocado, sliced
- 1 tbsp olive oil
- 2 eggs

1 Spread the cream cheese over both halves of the toasted bagels. Add the salmon to the bottom halves, then top with the avocado, season well.

2 Heat the oil in a non-stick frying pan. When hot, crack in the eggs, season and cook for 2–3 mins until the white is set and starting to crisp up around the edges. Sit the eggs on top of each bagel base, top with the other half of the bagel and serve.

Nutrition per serving
Kcals 681 • fat 36g • saturates 10g • carbs 53g • sugars 6g • fibre 6g • protein 33g • salt 2.4g

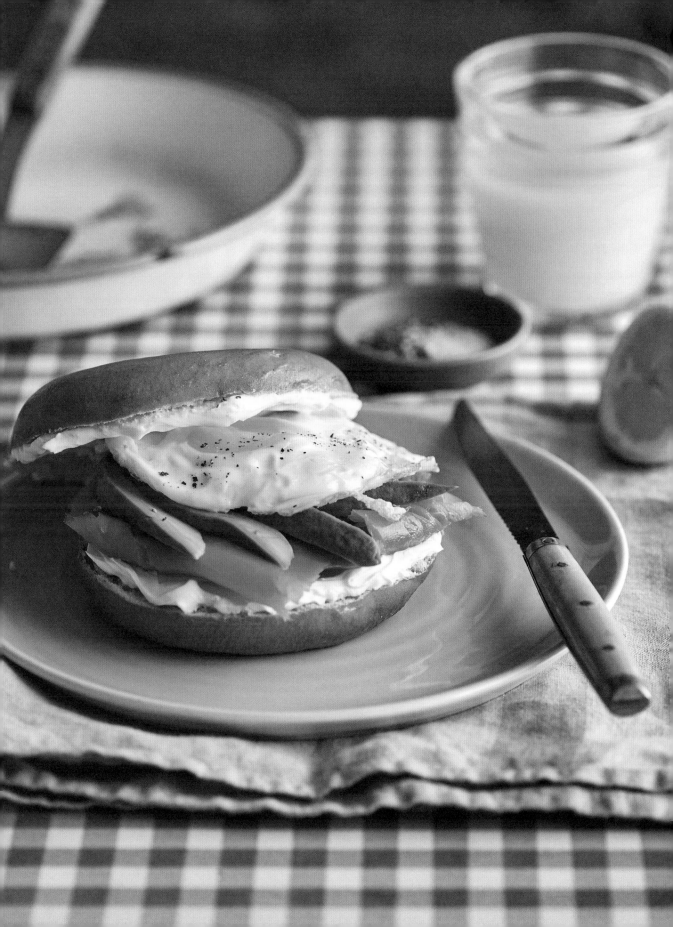

Sausage & egg baps

Give the humble sausage sarnie the brunch treatment by serving it in buns with a piquant tomato salsa or ketchup.

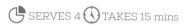 SERVES 4 ⏱ TAKES 15 mins

- 12 Cumberland sausages
- 1 tsp vegetable oil
- 4 large eggs
- 4 large soft white or wholemeal baps
- 4 tbsp tomato salsa

1 Squeeze the sausagemeat from the skins and shape into 4 flat patties. Heat the oil in a large frying pan. Cook the patties for 4 mins each side, squashing them down with the back of a spatula, until crisp and golden on both sides. Remove from the pan and keep warm.

2 Heat the grill. Crack the eggs into the pan and cook to your liking. Meanwhile, slice open the baps and lightly toast, cut-side up, under the grill. Add a spoonful of the salsa to each bap, then a sausage patty, then top with a fried egg.

Nutrition per serving
Kcals 747 • fat 49g • saturates 17g • carbs 45g • sugars 14g • fibre 2g • protein 31g • salt 4.6g

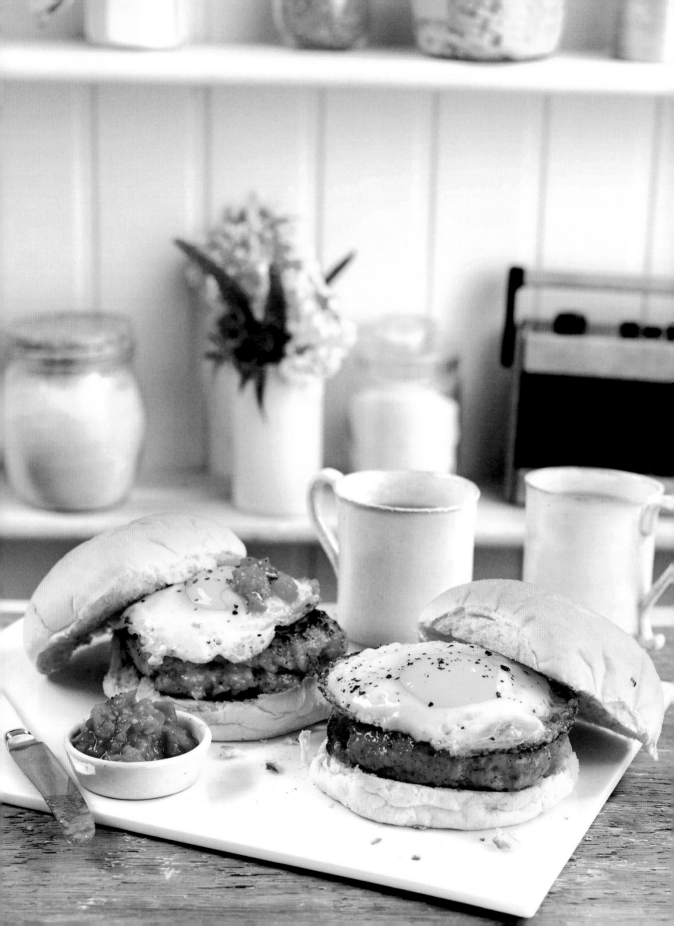

Cinnamon cashew spread with apple slices

This simple spread makes a handy vegan snack. Spread it on apple rounds for an easy way to get one of your 5-a-day.

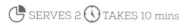 SERVES 2 TAKES 10 mins

- 50g unroasted cashew nuts
- 1 tbsp coconut oil
- ½ tsp cinnamon
- 2 apples, sliced straight across into rounds
- 2 generous lemon wedges, for squeezing over

1 Pour boiling water over the cashew nuts in a small bowl to cover, and leave for 2–3 mins so they soften a little. Drain, then return to the bowl. Add the coconut oil and cinnamon and blitz with a stick blender to chop the nuts into a rough paste. Serve with the apples slices and lemon wedges.

Nutrition per serving
Kcals 239 • fat 18g • saturates 7g • carbs 12g • sugars 9g • fibre 3g • protein 6g • salt 0g

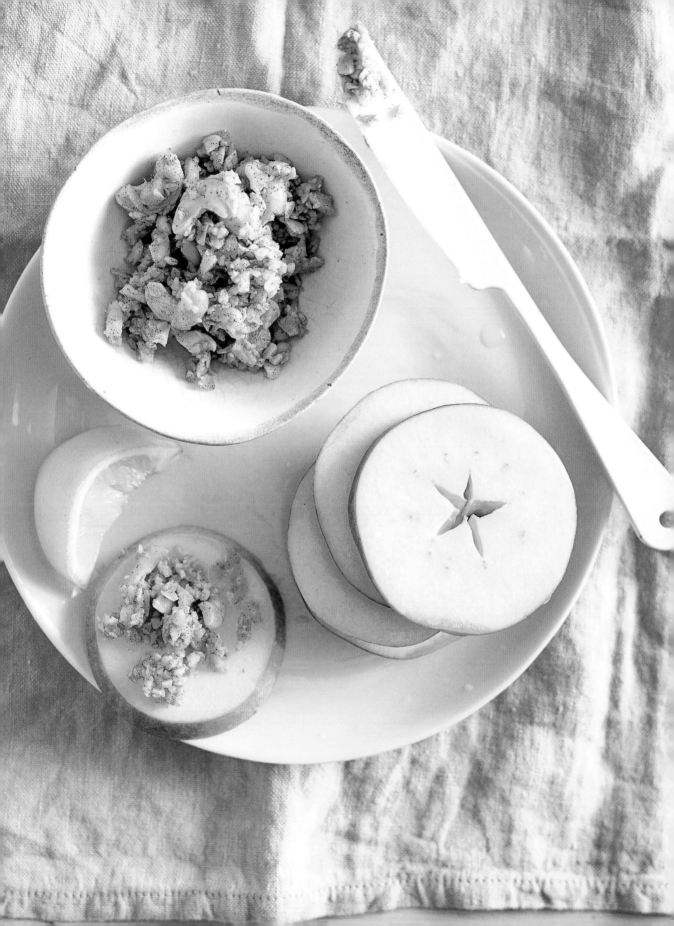

Breakfast knickerbocker glory

A summer sundae, but not as you know it … This brunch-friendly layered treat contains sorbet, frozen yogurt, fresh blueberries and granola.

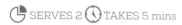 SERVES 2 TAKES 5 mins

- 4 tbsp granola
- fresh fruit, we used a handful of blueberries and 1 small ripe mango, peeled and sliced
- 2 tbsp clear honey or maple syrup
- 2–4 scoops raspberry sorbet
- 2 scoops frozen natural yogurt

1 Divide the granola between 2 sundae glasses (save a little for the top). Layer the berries, honey, sorbet, mango and frozen yogurt on top, then finish with a final sprinkling of granola, and a drizzle of honey.

Nutrition per serving
Kcals 414 • fat 9g • saturates 3g • carbs 74g • sugars 59g • fibre 4g • protein 7g • salt 0.2g

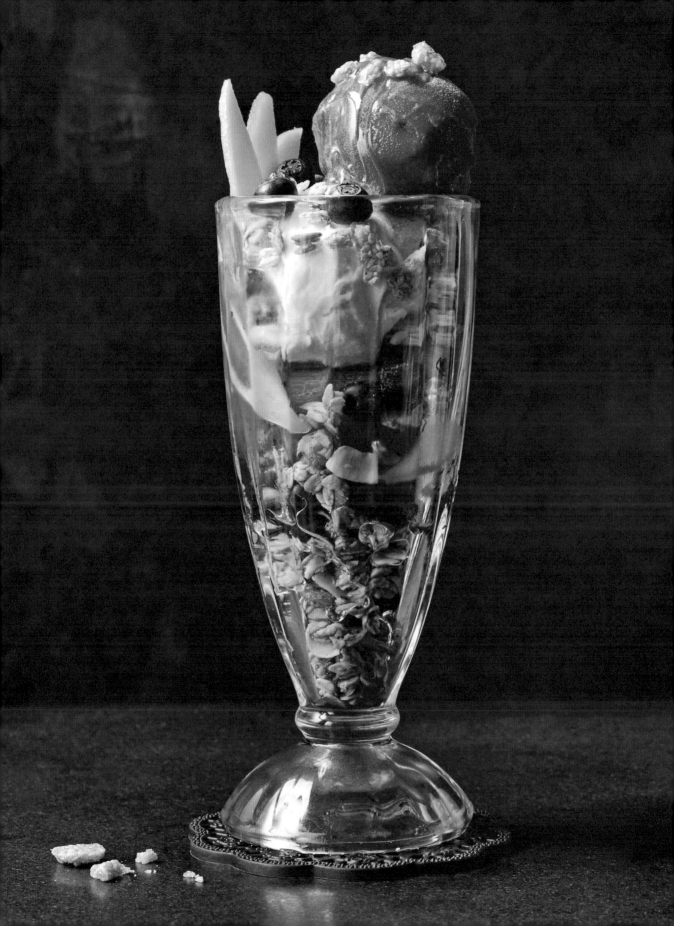

Avocado & strawberry smoothie

A creamy breakfast-friendly blend that's high in calcium and low in calories.

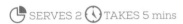 SERVES 2 TAKES 5 mins

- ½ avocado, stoned, peeled and cut into chunks
- 150g strawberries, halved
- 4 tbsp low-fat natural yogurt
- 200ml semi-skimmed milk
- lemon or lime juice, to taste

1 Put all the ingredients in a blender and whizz until smooth. If the consistency is too thick, add a little water.

Nutrition per serving
Kcals 197 • fat 11g • saturates 3g • carbs 15g • sugars 15g • fibre 3g • protein 9g • salt 0.3g

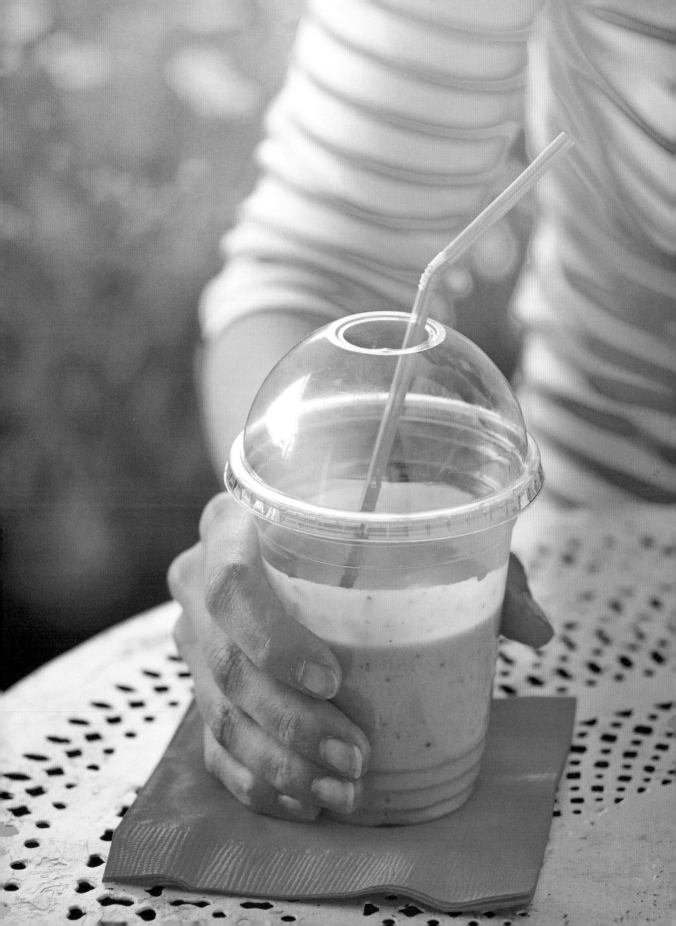

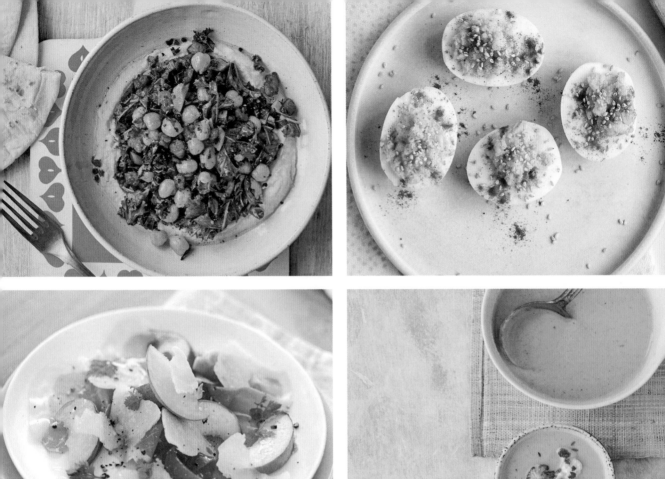

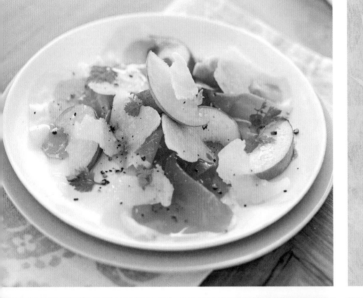

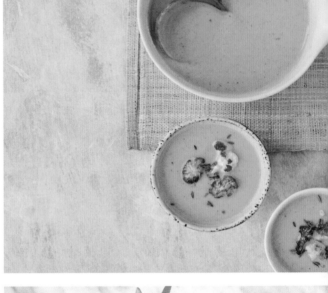

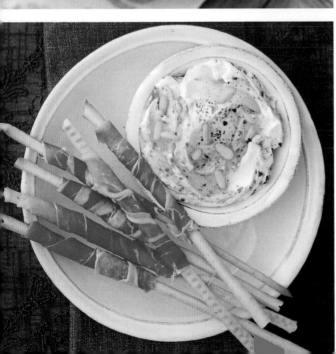

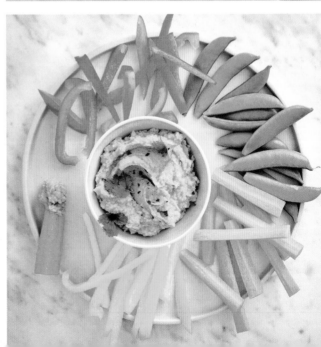

CHAPTER 2: STARTERS

If you're going in for a full three-course menu, it's often the starter that can cause the most stress. What to cook? How to time it perfectly around the main course? Have no fear, the recipes in this chapter are all super simple to put together and will add hardly any work at all to your dinner prep. There's something in here for every occasion, season and diet. These recipes are all super easy and you'll want to keep making them time and time again.

Creamy pesto with prosciutto dippers

Barely any more effort than opening a bag of crisps – and your party guests will be so much more impressed with this.

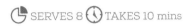 SERVES 8 ⏱ TAKES 10 mins

- 300g tub light soft cheese
- 2 tbsp basil pesto
- 140g pack grissini (bread sticks)
- 90g pack prosciutto
- 1 tbsp pine nuts
- extra virgin olive oil, for drizzling

1 Mix the soft cheese with the basil pesto. Take the pack of grissini (bread sticks) and halve each one. Cut the prosciutto into strips and wrap around the end of each grissini. Serve alongside the pesto dip. Scatter the pine nuts over the dip and drizzle with extra virgin olive oil before serving.

Nutrition per serving
Kcals 179 • fat 10g • saturates 4g • carbs 14g • sugars 3g • fibre 1g • protein 9g • salt 1.22g

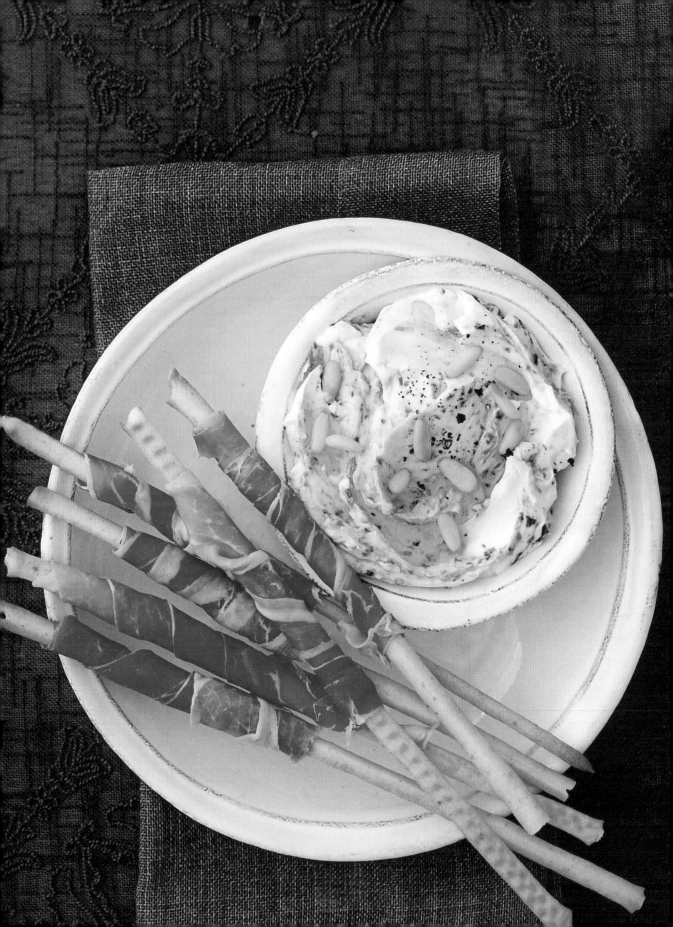

Faux gras

With only 2 ingredients, this is the easiest parfait you'll ever make. If you have a smoothie bullet blender, it'll give you the most velvety result.

SERVES 6-8 TAKES 25 mins plus chilling

- 100g butter, softened
- 300g organic chicken or duck livers, trimmed, cleaned and patted dry
- sliced brioche or sourdough, to serve
- cornichons, to serve
- chutney, to serve

1 Heat 50g butter in a frying pan until sizzling, add the livers and fry for 4 mins until coloured on the outside and slightly pink in the middle. Leave to cool, then tip the contents of the pan into a food processor or a smoothie bullet blender. Season generously with salt and add the remaining butter. Blitz until you have a smooth purée, then scrape into a container, smooth over the top and place in the fridge to chill for at least 2 hrs. Can be made a day ahead.

2 To serve, griddle slices of brioche or sourdough, and tip some cornichons and chutney into small pots. Put a large spoon in a cup of hot water. As if serving ice cream, scoop a spoonful of the faux gras onto each plate, dipping the spoon into the water after each scoop. Sprinkle a few salt flakes over each scoop and serve with the toasts, cornichons and chutney.

Nutrition per serving (8)
Kcals 127 • fat 11g • saturates 7g • carbs 0g • sugars 0g • fibre 0g • protein 7g • salt 0.3g

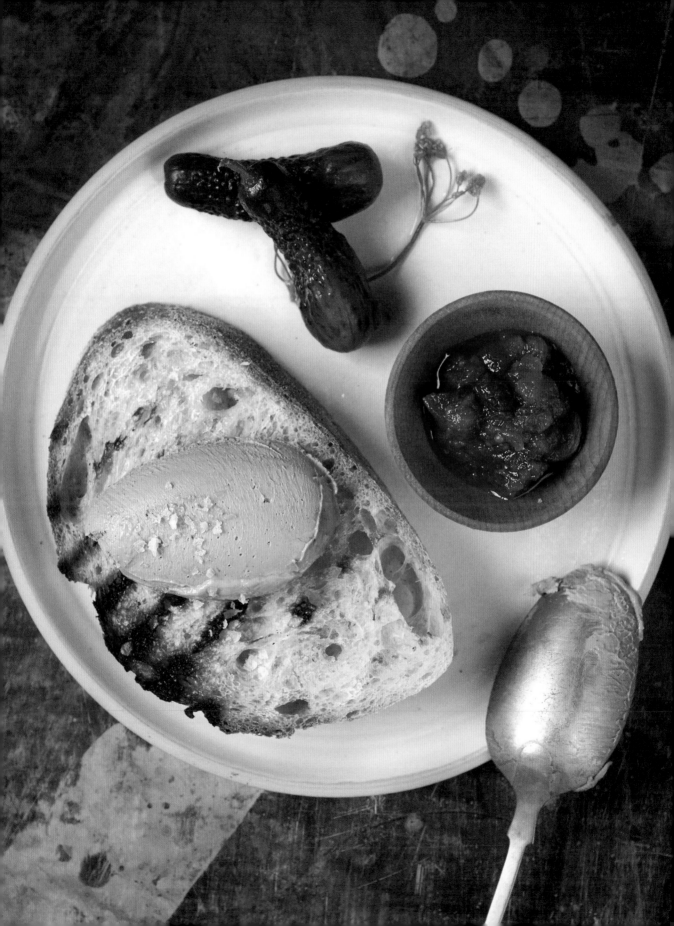

Ajo blanco

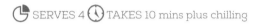

Chilled almond soup makes a refreshing starter and only has 4 ingredients for an authentic Spanish taste.

SERVES 4 · TAKES 10 mins plus chilling

- 200g blanched almonds
- 50ml extra virgin olive oil
- 1 garlic clove (if you like garlic, try with 1½ cloves)
- 1½ tbsp red wine vinegar

1 Blend all the ingredients together with 350ml water and 1 tsp salt.
2 Let the soup cool in the fridge for 1 hour or so, then serve with a drizzle of oil and some black pepper.

Nutrition per serving
Kcals 265 · fat 25g · saturates 3g · carbs 2g · sugars 1g · fibre 0g · protein 8g · salt 0.8g

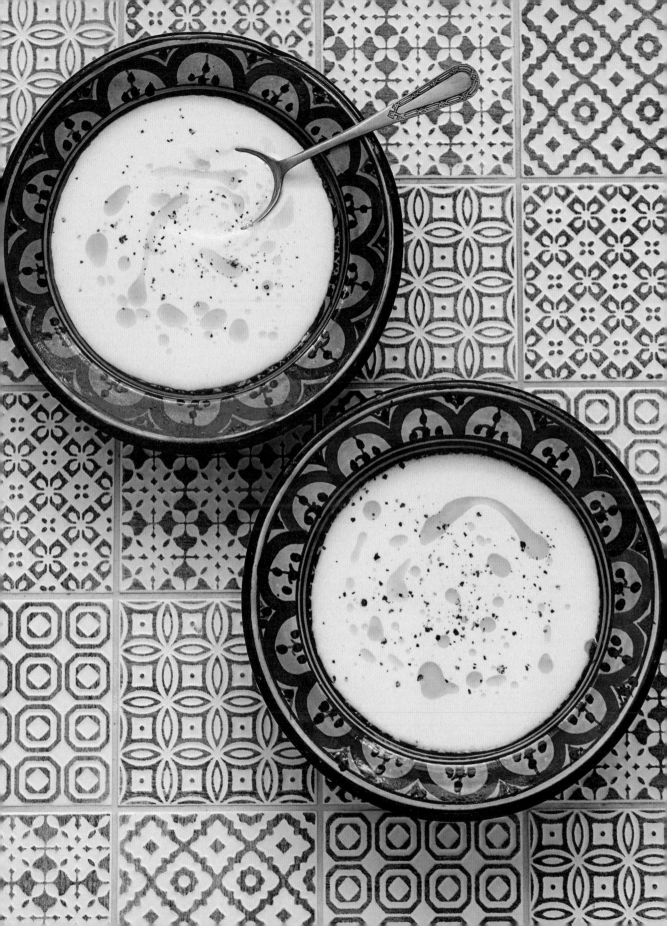

Chorizo hummus bowl

Add chorizo and kale to hummus for a dish that's packed with protein and flavour. Drizzle over olive oil and serve with flatbread for a lunch for one or a sharing starter for a crowd.

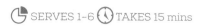 SERVES 1-6 TAKES 15 mins

- 400g can chickpeas
- 2 tbsp olive oil
- ¼ lemon, juiced
- 1–2 small cooking chorizo, chopped
- 2 handfuls chopped kale
- flatbread, to serve

1 Warm the chickpeas in a microwave or frying pan in their liquid. Drain and reserve the liquid. Tip half the chickpeas into a small food processor with 1 tbsp oil, the lemon juice and a splash of the liquid from the chickpea can and whizz to a paste. Season.

2 Put the chorizo in a small frying pan and cook over a low heat until it starts to release its oils, then turn up the heat and continue cooking until the chorizo starts to crisp. Add the remaining chickpeas and stir for a couple of mins. Stir in the kale and cook until it wilts.

3 Spoon the warm hummus into a bowl and tip the chorizo, chickpeas and kale on top. Drizzle over the remaining oil, season well and serve with flatbread for scooping up.

Nutrition per serving (for one)
Kcals 758 • fat 47g • saturates 10g • carbs 43g • sugars 2g • fibre 14g • protein 33g • salt 2g

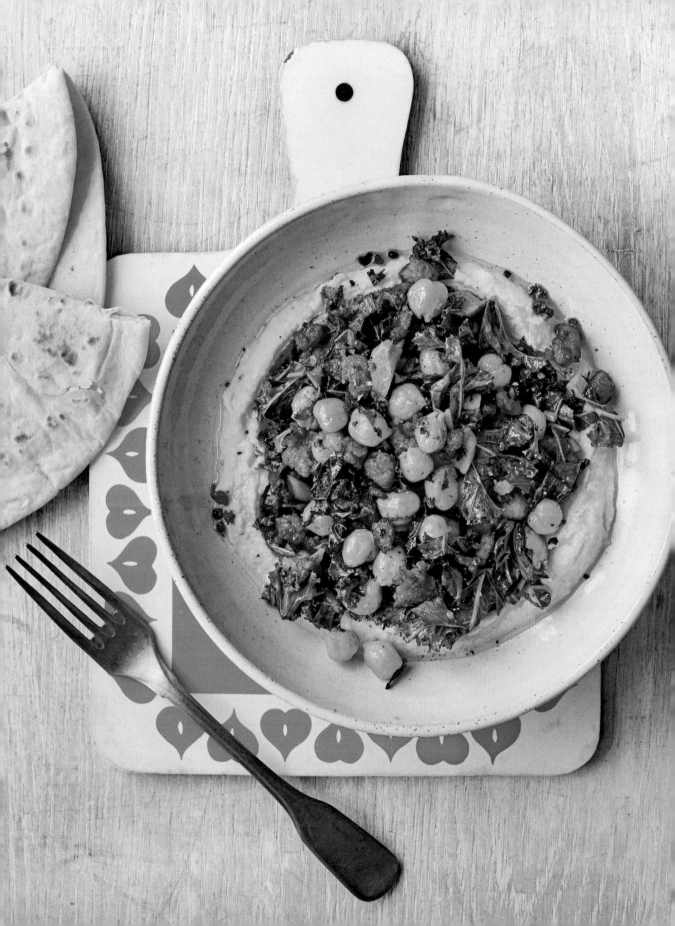

Avocado hummus

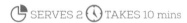

Get all 5 of your 5-a-day with this healthy, low-calorie, vegan recipe that works as lunch or a starter. Enjoy deliciously creamy hummus made with avocado.

SERVES 2   TAKES 10 mins

- 1 avocado, halved, stoned and peeled
- 210g chickpeas, drained
- pinch chilli flakes, plus extra to serve
- 1 lime, juiced
- handful coriander leaves

1 Blitz together the avocado, chickpeas, chilli flakes and lime juice, and season to taste. Top the hummus with the coriander leaves and a few more chilli flakes, and serve with veggies for dipping.

Nutrition per serving
Kcals 335 • fat 17g • saturates 3g • carbs 28g • sugars 15g • fibre 15g • protein 10g • salt 0.2g

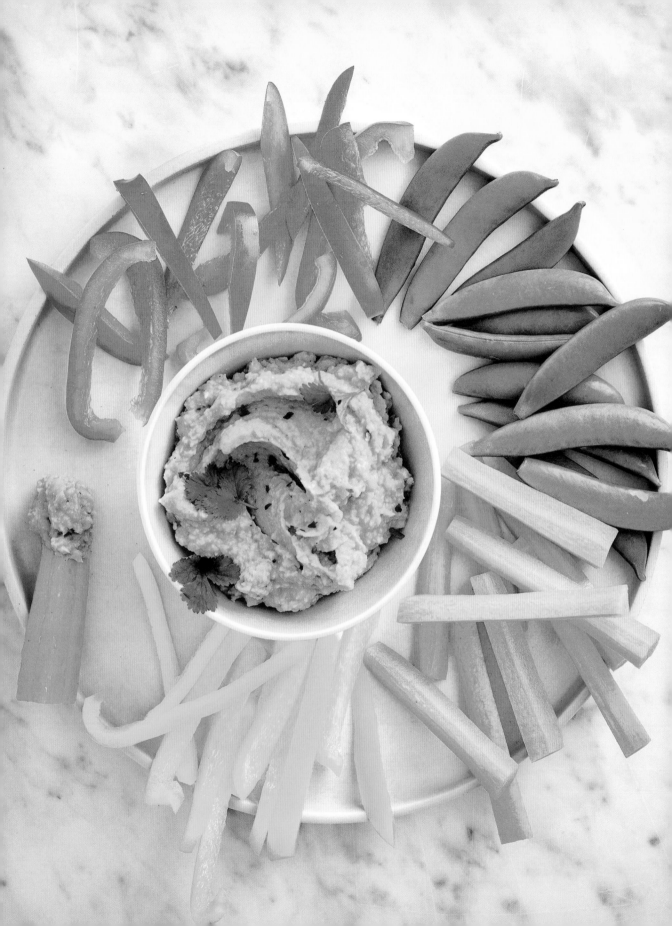

Miso & sesame eggs

Perfect as a snack or a dinner party nibble, miso adds a deep savoury flavour to these low-calorie eggs. Try them served on salad for a quick and tasty lunch, or as a starter.

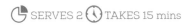 SERVES 2 TAKES 15 mins

- 2 large eggs
- 1 tsp white miso
- 2 tsp toasted sesame seeds
- a little smoked paprika

1 Hard-boil the eggs for 10 mins then cool under running water. When cool enough to handle, carefully remove the shells.
2 Halve the eggs and scoop out their yolks into a small bowl. Add the miso and mash together, adding a dash of water to give a creamy consistency. Spoon back into the eggs and scatter with the seeds, then sprinkle over the paprika. Eat straight away or keep in the fridge for up to 2 days.

Nutrition per serving
Kcals 121 • fat 8g • saturates 2g • carbs 1g • sugars 0.1g • fibre 1g • protein 10g • salt 0.48g

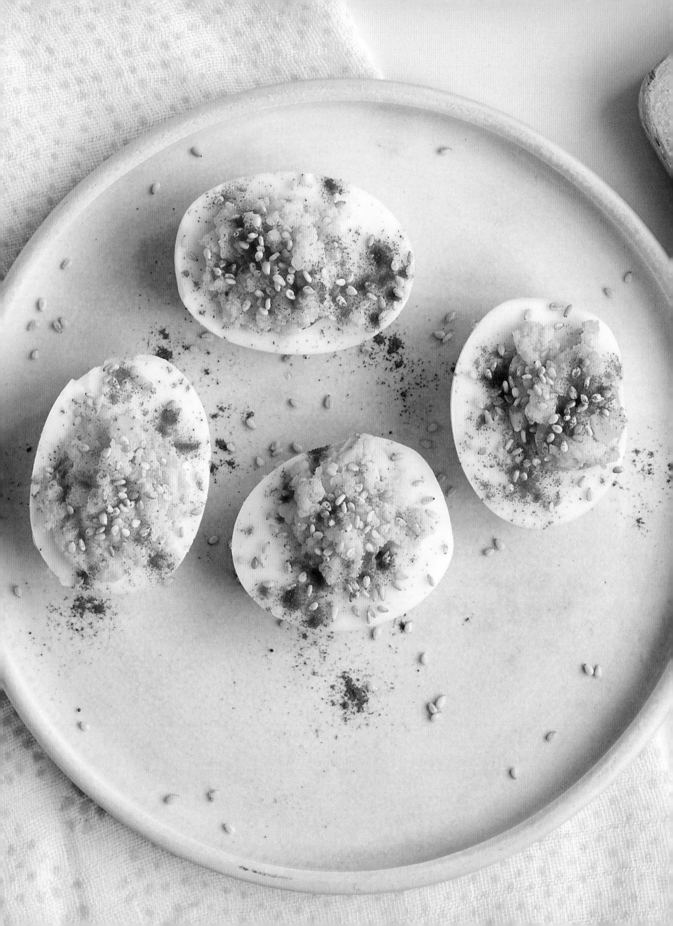

Cheese & tarragon stuffed mushrooms

Make this speedy, cheesy veggie treat for a light supper, or starter. It only needs 5 ingredients and you can have it on the table in 15 minutes.

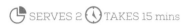 SERVES 2 TAKES 15 mins

- 4 large Portobello mushrooms
- 3 tbsp ricotta
- 30g parmesan (or vegetarian) alternative, grated
- 30g grated mozzarella or cheddar
- 1 tbsp tarragon leaves (optional)

1 Heat the grill to high. Remove the central stalks of the mushrooms, season and place on a baking tray. Mix the cheeses and tarragon together and season. Spoon the cheese mixture onto the mushrooms and grill for 8–10 mins, or until bubbling and oozy.

2 Remove from the tray with a spatula, season and serve with a rocket salad.

Nutrition per serving
Kcals 216 • fat 13g • saturates 8g • carbs 5g • sugars 5g • fibre 3g • protein 17g • salt 0.6g

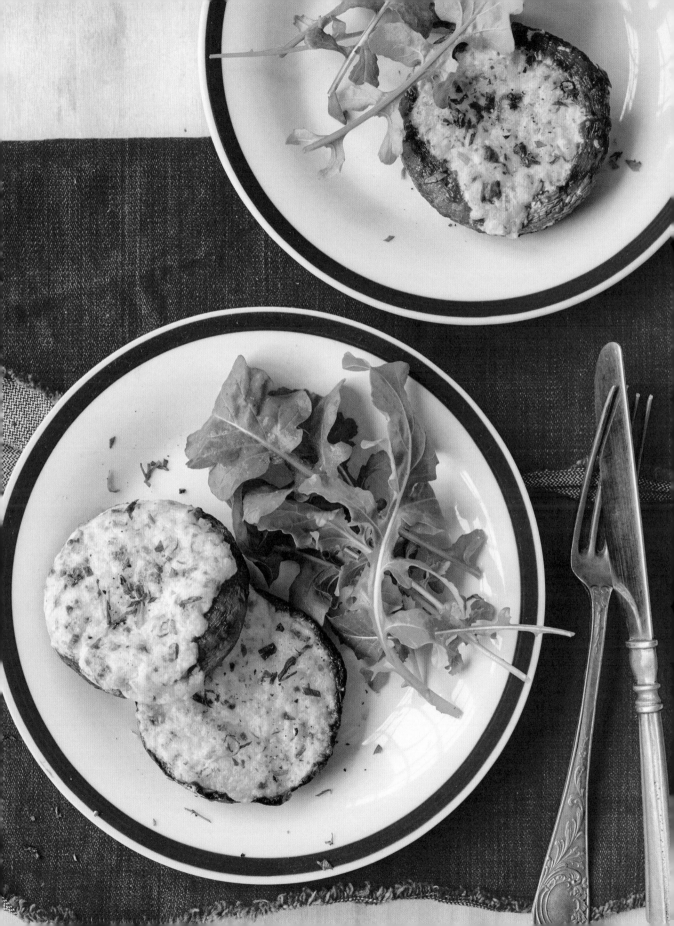

Parma ham & peach plates

Take a trip to the deli to make this easy but impressive summer starter for two.

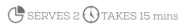 SERVES 2 TAKES 15 mins

- 6 slices Parma ham
- 1 peach, halved and stoned
- 25g chunk parmesan
- 1 tbsp extra virgin olive oil
- few chervil sprigs, to serve

1 Arrange 3 slices of the ham on each plate. Slice each peach half into 6 wedges, then scatter these over the ham.
2 Shave the parmesan over both plates, then drizzle with a little oil. Scatter with cracked black pepper and chervil, then serve.

Nutrition per serving
Kcals 215 • fat 15g • saturates 5g • carbs 4g • sugars 4g • fibre 1g • protein 17g • salt 2.4g

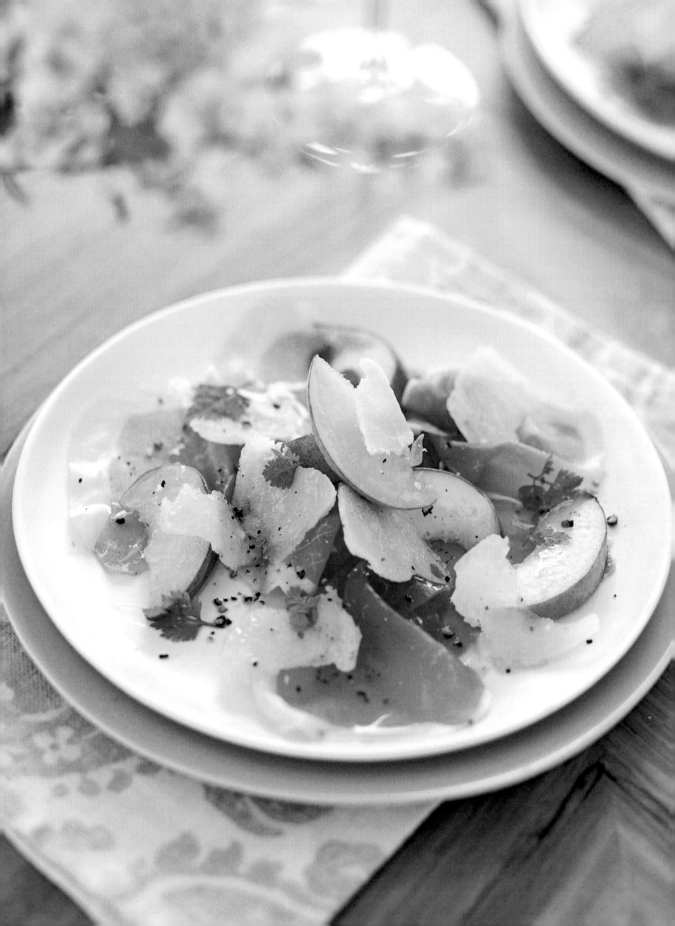

Smoked mackerel pâté with cucumber

This impressive and delicately flavoured starter is perfect for dinner parties without splashing the cash. Make-ahead, easy-to-do and no cooking required.

SERVES 6 TAKES 30 mins plus chilling

- 1 pack smoked mackerel (about 200g)
- 250g tub cream cheese
- 2 lemons, 1 zested, both juiced
- small pack dill, half roughly chopped, half fronds picked
- 1 cucumber
- 4 tbsp olive oil, plus extra to drizzle

1 Peel and flake the mackerel and tip into a small blender with the cream cheese, lemon zest and half the lemon juice, and pulse to make a pâté. Add the chopped dill and pulse again to mix.

2 Tip the mixture into a plastic piping bag or sandwich bag, cut off the end and pipe 6 thick cylinders of the pâté onto a baking tray and put in the freezer to harden for about 1 hr.

3 Remove a strip of peel from the cucumber – it's easiest with a swivel peeler, but a normal one also works – then peel 12 neat ribbons off the cucumber. Do not throw away any of the seeds or the peelings. Dice any remaining flesh, cover and put in the fridge ready to use later. Use the neat ribbons to wrap around the pâté and put in the fridge. Can be made up to 1 day ahead.

4 Tip the cucumber peelings and seeds into a blender or smoothie maker with the rest of the lemon juice, the olive oil and some seasoning. Blitz to make a thick dressing, then chill. Can be made 1 day ahead and kept in the fridge.

5 To serve, pour a little dressing onto each plate, sit a cucumber-wrapped pâté on top, neatly scatter the diced cucumber and dill fronds, and drizzle over more olive oil.

Nutrition per serving
Kcals 283 • fat 26g • saturates 9g • carbs 2g • sugars 2g • fibre 1g • protein 10g • salt 0.9g

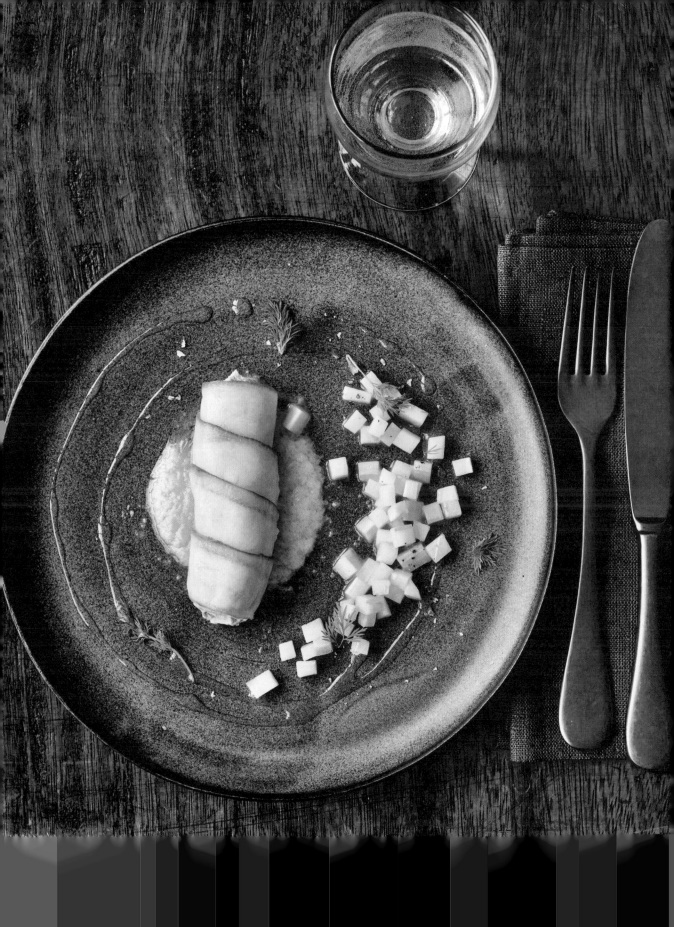

Smoked salmon terrine

A show-stopping layered fish centrepiece with cream cheese and lemon filling, flavoured with chives.

MAKES 1 TERRINE (CUTS INTO 8–10 SLICES) · TAKES 50 mins plus overnight chilling

- 600g smoked salmon slices
- 600g cream cheese
- 150ml double cream
- zest and juice 1 lemon and thin wedges, to serve
- 2 tbsp finely snipped chive
- a little oil, for greasing

1 Grease a loaf tin, a 900g one is ideal but you can use one slightly smaller or bigger. Line with cling film, then cover just the base with one layer of smoked salmon slices, trimmed to fit neatly.

2 Whizz the cream cheese, cream, lemon zest and juice together in a food processor to combine. Scrape out and stir in the chives with some seasoning. Spread an 8th of the cream cheese mixture over as evenly as you can. Top with a layer of salmon slices. Repeat with the cream cheese and salmon – you should be able to do 7 layers of cream cheese. (By starting with just an 8th of the mixture, it means as the tin widens you'll have enough to put a bit more as you go further up creating even layers.) Finish with a last layer of salmon (and treat yourself to a smoked salmon sarnie with any trimmings!) Cover with cling film, pressing down gently, then chill overnight.

3 To serve, turn onto a platter and gently peel off the cling film. Serve with rocket salad and melba toast.

Nutrition per serving (10)
Kcals 339 • fat 29g • saturates 16g • carbs 2g • sugars 2g • fibre 0.1g • protein 17g • salt 2.2g

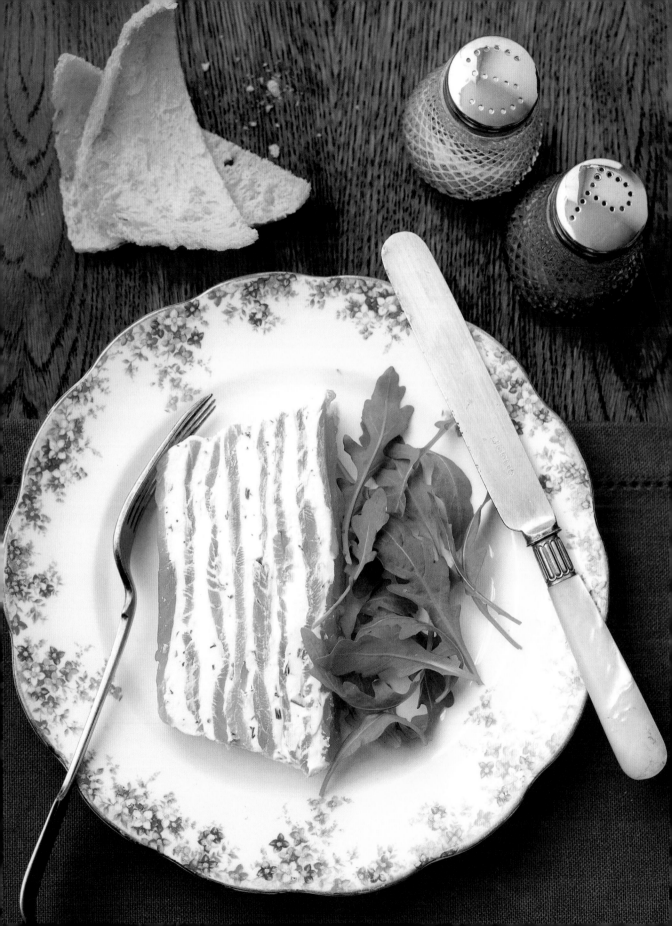

Curried cauliflower & lentil soup

Take one cauliflower and blend with red lentils, fennel seeds, curry paste and lemon juice to be rewarded with this warming, hearty soup.

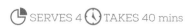 SERVES 4 TAKES 40 mins

- 1 cauliflower
- 1½ tbsp oil
- 2 tsp fennel seeds
- 150g red lentils
- 3 tbsp curry paste of your choice
- ½ lemon, juiced

1 Remove the outer leaves from the cauliflower, cut off the stalk and roughly chop, then cut the head into small florets. Toss a quarter of the florets in 1 tbsp oil and 1 tsp of the fennel seeds, season well, then tip into a roasting tin and set aside.

2 Heat oven to 220C/200C fan/gas 7. Heat ½ tbsp oil in a saucepan over a medium heat and add the remaining fennel seeds, toast for 2 mins, then add the lentils and the remaining cauliflower. Stir in the curry paste, then add 1 litre water and bring to the boil. Simmer for 25 mins until the cauliflower is tender and the lentils are cooked through.

3 Meanwhile, put the roasting tin of cauliflower in the oven and cook for 20 mins until crisp and slightly charred. Tip the soup mixture into a food processor and blitz until smooth, tip back into the pan to warm through, adding the lemon juice and a little water if it's too thick. Tip into bowls and top with the crispy cauliflower and fennel seeds to serve.

Nutrition per serving
Kcals 242 • fat 8g • saturates 1g • carbs 27g • sugars 5g • fibre 6g • protein 13g • salt 0.5g

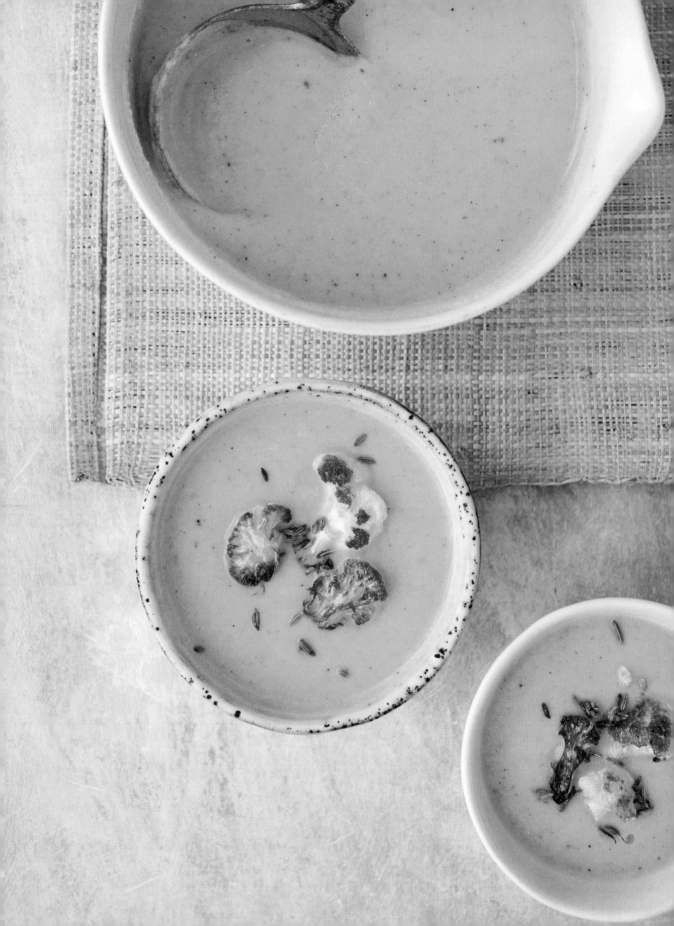

Cucumber, pea & lettuce soup

Treat as a healthy lunch or vegetarian starter, this simple and refreshing vibrant green soup is low in calories and features 3 of your 5-a-day.

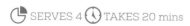 SERVES 4 TAKES 20 mins

- 1 tsp rapeseed oil
- small bunch spring onions, roughly chopped
- 1 cucumber, roughly chopped
- 1 large round lettuce, roughly chopped
- 225g frozen peas
- 4 tsp vegetable bouillon

1 Boil 1.4 litres water in a kettle. Heat the oil in a large non-stick frying pan and cook the spring onions for 5 mins, stirring frequently, or until softened. Add the cucumber, lettuce and peas, then pour in the boiled water. Stir in the bouillon, cover and simmer for 10 mins or until the vegetables are soft but still bright green.
2 Blitz the mixture with a hand blender until smooth. Serve hot or cold, topped with yogurt (if you like) and with rye bread alongside.

Nutrition per serving
Kcals 156 • fat 3g • saturates 0g • carbs 21g • sugars 7g • fibre 7g • protein 8g • salt 0.6g

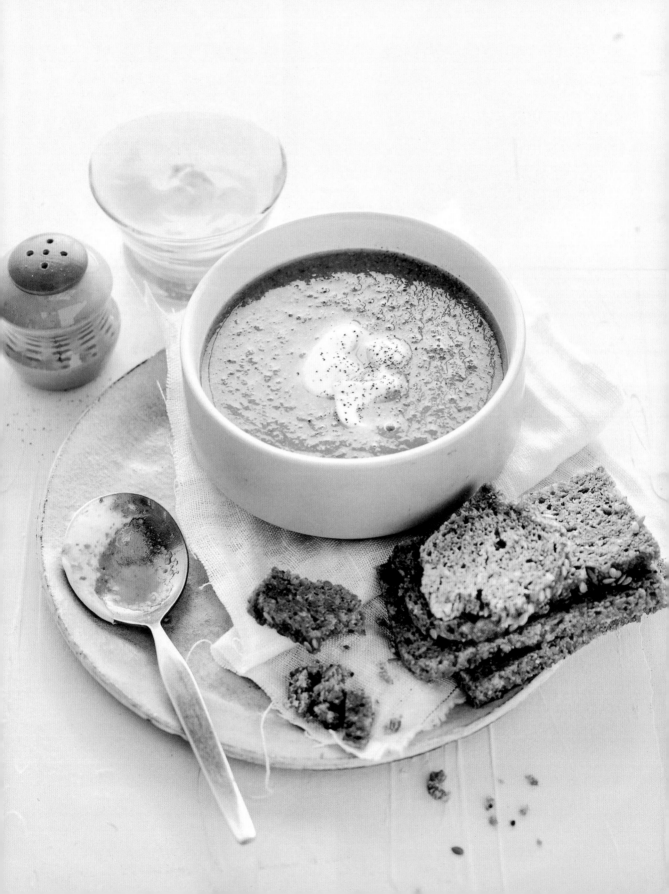

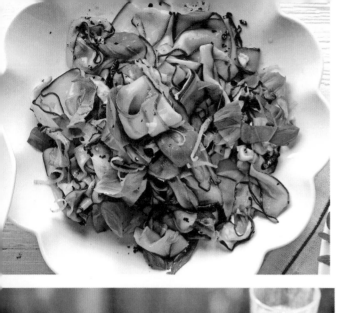

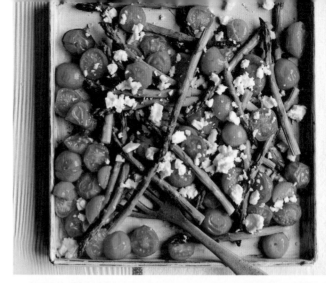

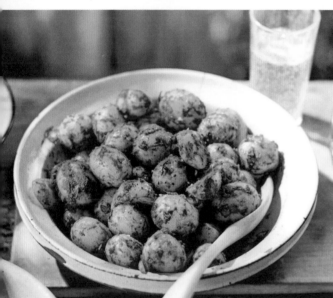

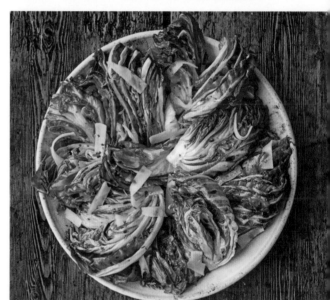

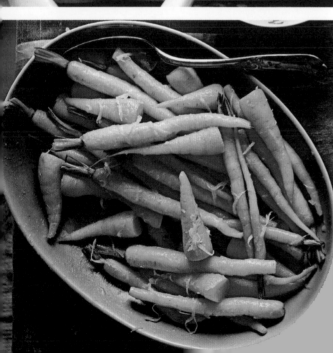

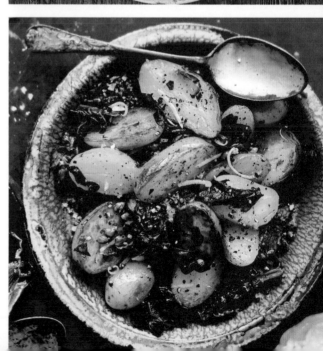

CHAPTER 3: SIDES

Vegetables and side dishes often get less love than they deserve, but it's amazing how delicious they can be when you put together a handful of interesting ingredients. Forget boiled carrots or peas, try our Pea-camole, a smashed-up cross between mushy peas and guacamole. Or how about our Ginger & orange glazed baby carrots for a zingy addition to your Sunday roast. Some of these recipes are so gorgeous they could work in a big bowl as a main course – the Butter bean, cucumber & radish salad would make a lovely light summer's day dinner. Give it a go.

Griddled baby gems with balsamic & goat's cheese

Try a new way with lettuce and griddle your leaves on a high heat. Serve with vinaigrette and creamy cheese.

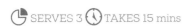 SERVES 3 TAKES 15 mins

- 4 Baby Gem lettuces, ends trimmed, quartered
- 3 tbsp olive oil
- 2 tbsp balsamic vinegar
- 1 tbsp clear honey
- 50g soft goat's cheese
- 50g pomegranate seeds

1 Put the lettuce in a bowl, drizzle with a little of the olive oil, then season. Place a griddle pan on a high heat. Griddle the lettuce for 30 secs-1 min per side or until slightly charred. Remove to a plate. Combine the balsamic vinegar and honey with some seasoning, then whisk in the remaining olive oil to make a dressing.

2 Drizzle the dressing over the lettuce. Crumble the goat's cheese on top of the salad and sprinkle with the pomegranate seeds.

Nutrition per serving
Kcals 233 • fat 17g • saturates 5g • carbs 14g • sugars 14g • fibre 4g • protein 6g • salt 0.3g

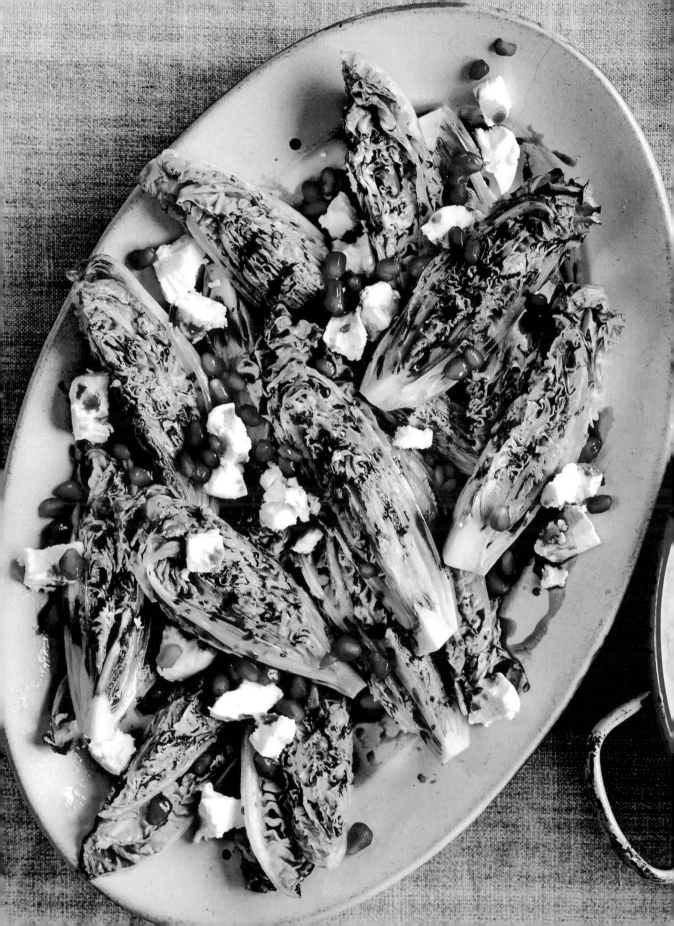

Warm lemony courgette salad

A healthy, vibrant salad of shaved courgette, citrus and basil. Serve as a gluten-free starter or side dish.

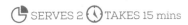 SERVES 2 ⏱ TAKES 15 mins

- 2 courgettes
- 1 tbsp olive oil
- zest 1 lemon, plus a squeeze of lemon
- 1 garlic clove, crushed
- ¼ small pack basil, roughly torn

1 Use a vegetable peeler to slice the courgettes into wide strips, discarding the central, seedy part. Heat the oil in a large frying pan, add the lemon zest and garlic, and fry over a medium heat for 1 min. Add the courgette strips and cook, stirring regularly, for a further 1–2 mins until the courgettes are slightly softened. Add a squeeze of lemon juice and toss the basil through.

Nutrition per serving
Kcals 71 • fat 6g • saturates 1g • carbs 2g • sugars 2g • fibre 1g • protein 2g • salt 0g

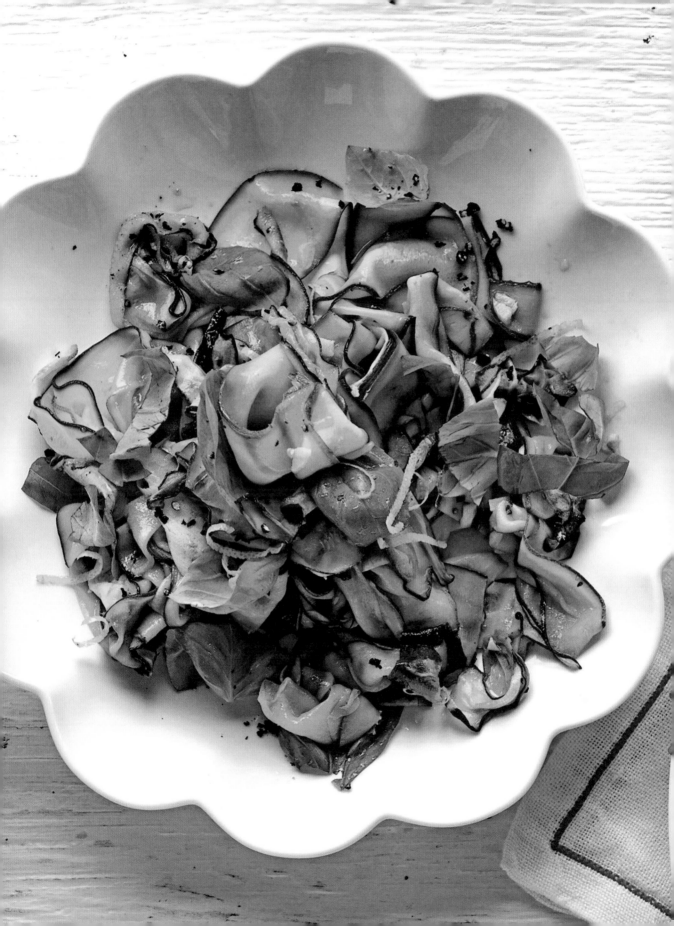

Cheesy leeks & ham

A low-carb side dish, perfect to serve alongside roast chicken and ready in just 25 mins.

SERVES 4 ⏲ TAKES 30 mins

- 8 small leeks, white part only
- 8 slices cooked ham
- 100g cheddar, grated
- 2 tbsp Dijon mustard
- 6 tbsp crème fraîche (full or half-fat)

1 Heat oven to 200C/180C fan/gas 6. Cook the leeks in a pan of boiling salted water for 4–5 mins or until just tender. Drain and cool under a cold tap to stop them from cooking any further, then drain again and pat dry on kitchen paper.

2 Wrap each leek in a slice of ham, then arrange, side-by-side, in a large baking dish. Mix the cheddar in a bowl with the Dijon mustard and crème fraîche, until well combined. Season to taste. Spread over the leeks, then bake for 15–20 mins until bubbling and golden brown. Serve at once with plenty of crusty bread to mop up the juices.

Nutrition per serving
Kcals 295 • fat 21g • saturates 12g • carbs 6g • sugars 0g • fibre 3g • protein 20g • salt 2g

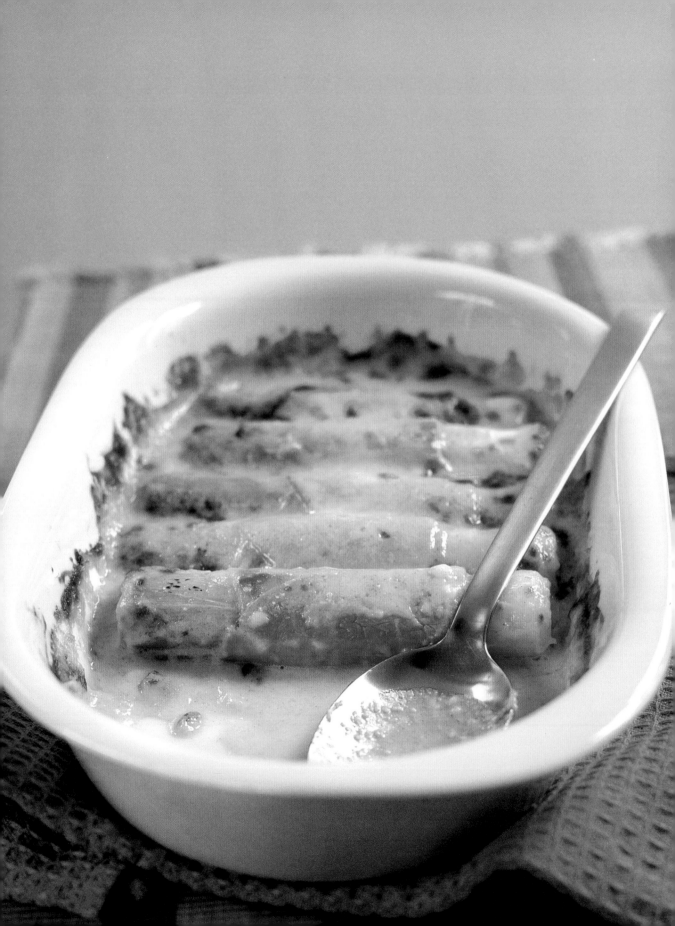

Roasted balsamic asparagus & cherry tomatoes

This simple vegetarian side dish can be served with meat, fish and veggie mains alike.

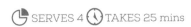 SERVES 4 TAKES 25 mins

- 350g asparagus spears, woody ends discarded
- 330g pack cherry tomatoes, halved
- 2 tbsp olive oil
- 1 tbsp balsamic vinegar
- 50g feta cheese, crumbled

1 Heat oven to 200C/180C fan/gas 6. Put the asparagus and cherry tomatoes on a baking tray. Drizzle over the olive oil and balsamic vinegar. Season, then toss everything together. Bake for 15 mins until the asparagus is cooked through. Serve topped with the feta.

Nutrition per serving
Kcals 120 • fat 9g • saturates 3g • carbs 5g • sugars 5g • fibre 3g • protein 5g • salt 0.5g

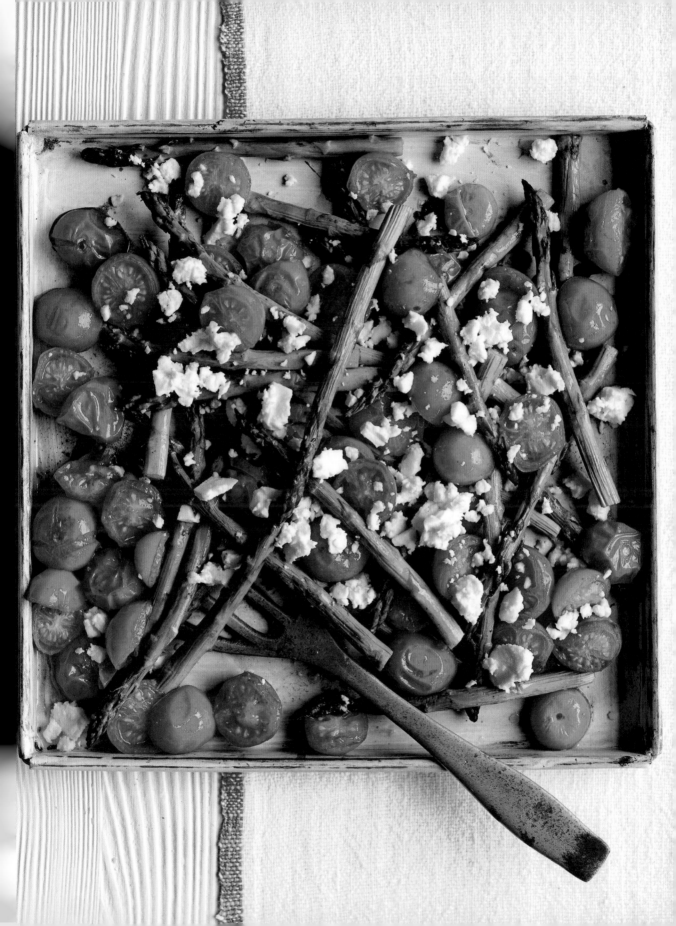

Salted maple roasted parsnips

Roast root vegetables with maple syrup and thyme leaves until soft and sticky, then serve as a side dish to a Sunday roast.

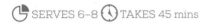 SERVES 6–8 ⏱ TAKES 45 mins

- 600g parsnips, peeled and quartered
- 2 tbsp vegetable oil
- 3 tbsp maple syrup
- 3 thyme sprigs, leaves picked

1 Heat oven to 220C/200C fan/gas 7. Put the parsnips in a large roasting tin with the oil, maple syrup, thyme leaves and some sea salt flakes. Roast for 35–40 mins until soft and sticky. Scatter over a few more sea salt flakes just before serving.

Nutrition per serving (8)
Kcals 97 • fat 3g • saturates 0g • carbs 15g • sugars 8g • fibre 4g • protein 1g • salt 0.3g

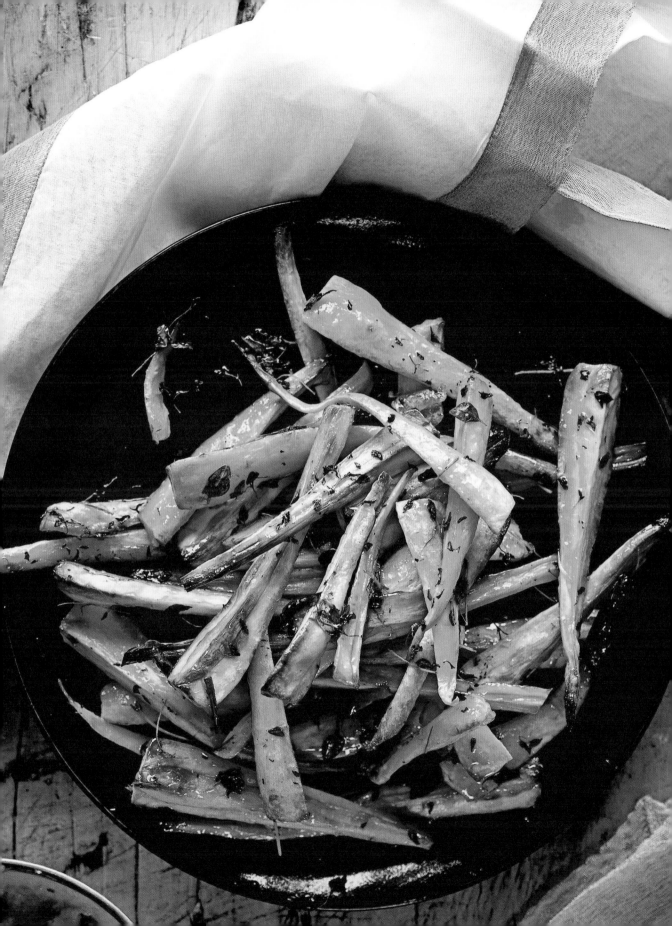

Ginger & orange glazed baby carrots

Pan-fry baby carrots with a zesty orange, ginger and honey sauce until golden and sticky for a flavourful root vegetable side.

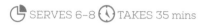 SERVES 6-8 TAKES 35 mins

- 900g baby carrots, washed and scrubbed
- 50g butter
- 25g piece ginger, peeled and finely grated
- 2 tbsp clear honey
- zest 1 orange

1 Bring a large pan of salted water to the boil and add the carrots. Simmer for 5 mins until slightly tender, then drain.
2 In a wide pan, heat the butter until melting, then add the carrots, ginger, honey and orange zest. Cook over a medium heat for 25–30 mins.
3 Turn the carrots gently in the pan every now and again until they start to go golden and sticky and all the sides are browning. Season well before serving.

Nutrition per serving
Kcals 101 • fat 6g • saturates 3g • carbs 10g • sugars 9g • fibre 4g • protein 1g • salt 0.4g

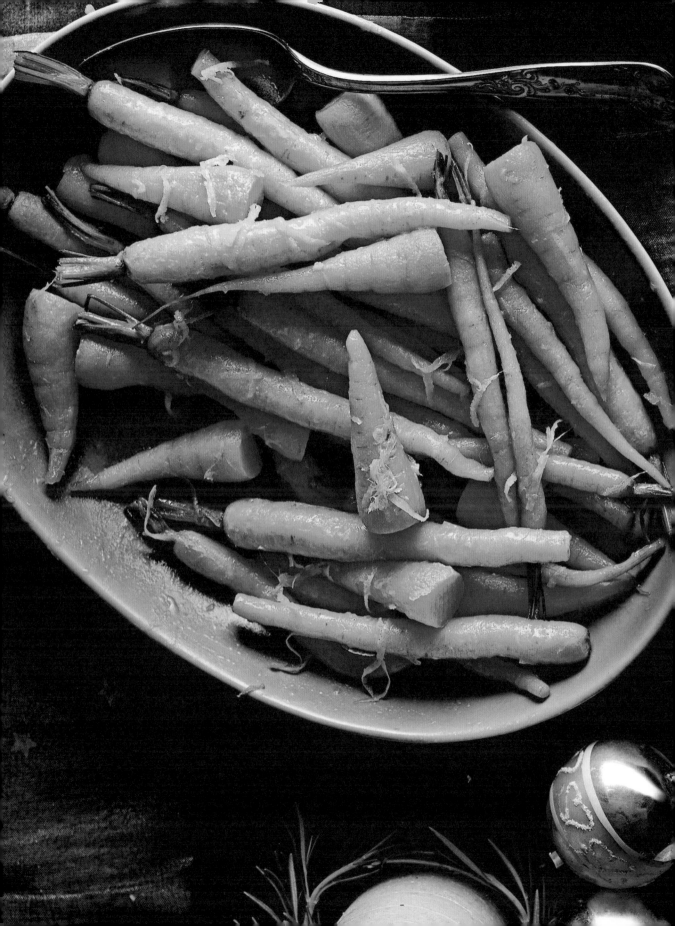

Courgetti with chilli, lemon, ricotta & mint

Dress your courgetti with fresh, zesty spring flavours. Use the best quality ricotta you can find in this simple, vibrant side dish.

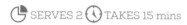 SERVES 2 TAKES 15 mins

- 2 courgettes (about 400g), ends trimmed and spiralized or peeled into thin noodles
- ½ red chilli, thinly sliced
- zest and juice ½ lemon
- ½ small pack mint, leaves picked
- 50g soft ricotta

1 Toss the courgetti in a bowl with the chilli, lemon juice, ¾ of the mint, some flaky sea salt and black pepper. Put onto a plate and garnish with the lemon zest, reserved mint and a dollop of the ricotta.

Nutrition per serving
Kcals 80 • fat 4g • saturates 2g • carbs 4g • sugars 4g • fibre 2g • protein 6g • salt 0.1g

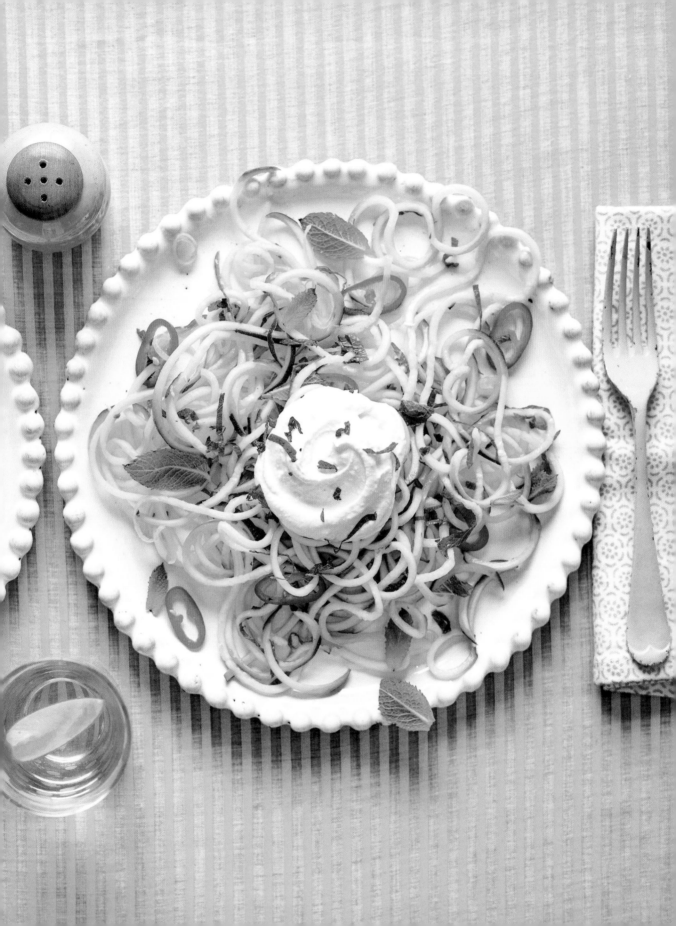

Pea-camole

Big kids love avocado, little kids love peas – and they add a good natural sweetness to this chilli-topping classic. It makes a handy vegan side dish too.

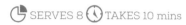 SERVES 8 TAKES 10 mins

- 200g frozen peas
- 2 ripe avocados, halved, stoned and peeled
- 2 limes, juiced
- small bunch coriander

1 Boil the kettle. Tip the peas into a mixing bowl and cover with about 2.5cm of boiling water. Leave for 5 mins to defrost, then drain well and tip back into the bowl.
2 Add the avocados with the lime juice and some salt, and mash everything together. Roughly chop the coriander and briefly mash through before serving.

Nutrition per serving
Kcals 93 • fat 7g • saturates 2g • carbs 3g • sugars 2g • fibre 3g • protein 2g • salt 0g

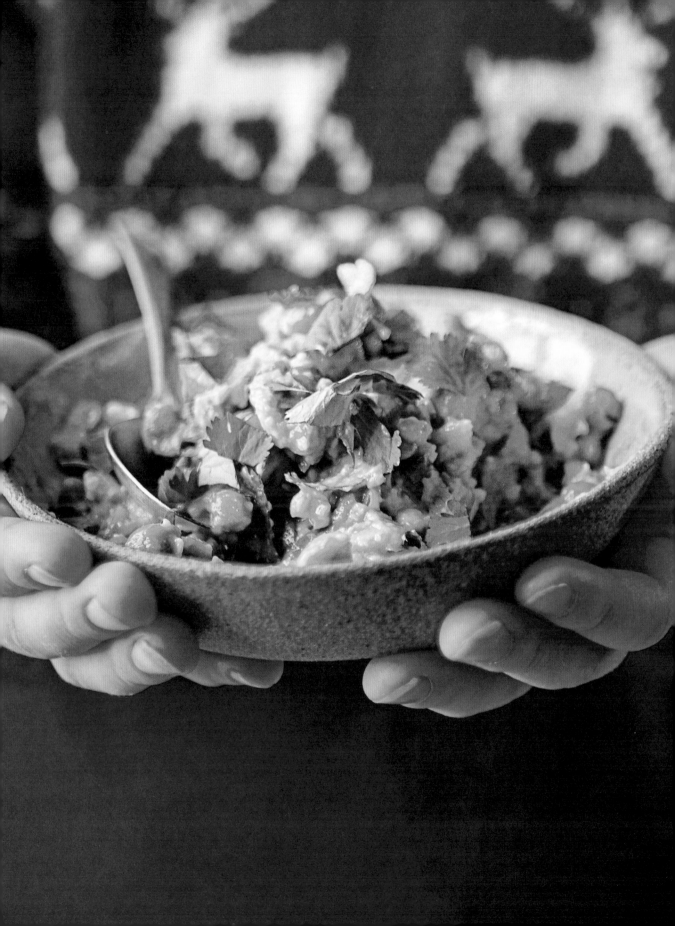

Easy creamy coleslaw

Give this classic side dish of crunchy grated vegetables a healthy makeover with a low-fat mustard mayonnaise dressing.

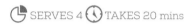 SERVES 4 · TAKES 20 mins

- ½ white cabbage, shredded
- 2 carrots, grated
- 4 spring onions, chopped
- 3 tbsp low-fat mayonnaise
- 1 tbsp wholegrain mustard

1 Put the cabbage, carrots, spring onions and sultanas in a large bowl and stir to combine.
2 Mix the mayonnaise with the mustard in another small bowl and drizzle over the veg. Fold everything together to coat in the creamy sauce, then season to taste.

OPTIONAL EXTRA
Try adding 2 tbsp sultanas or a handful of chopped pecans.

Nutrition per serving
Kcals 151 · fat 5g · saturates 1g · carbs 20g · sugars 14g · fibre 5g · protein 3g · salt 0.7g

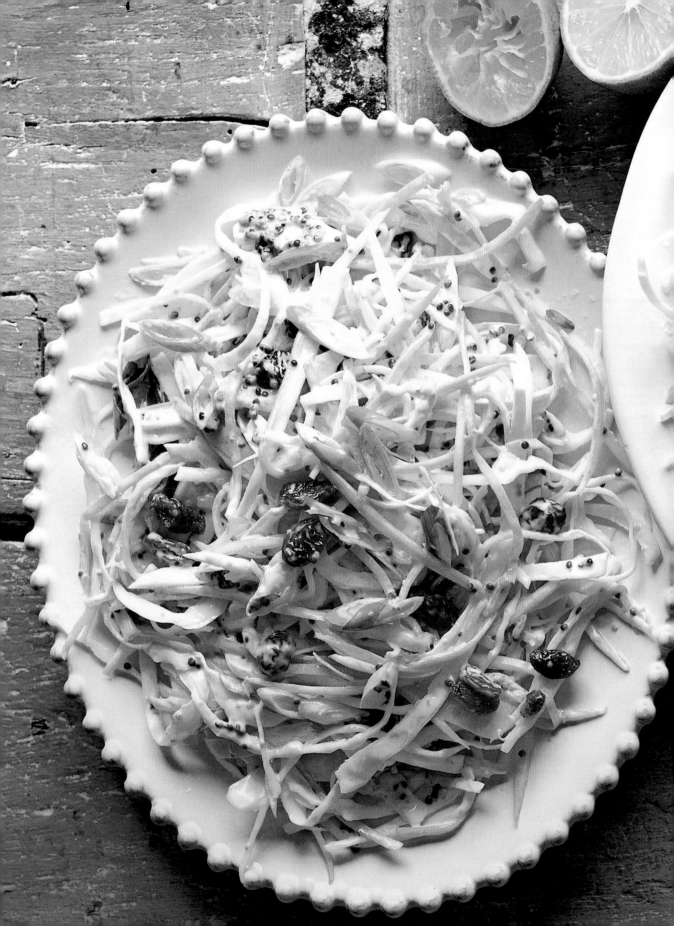

Butter bean, cucumber & radish salad

Crunch and freshness are the order of the day with this zesty, healthy side salad with pulses and herbs.

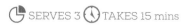 SERVES 3 TAKES 15 mins

- small bunch mint or parsley, chopped
- zest and juice ½ lemon
- 1 tbsp olive oil
- 2 x 400g cans butter beans, drained and rinsed
- 200g pack radishes, trimmed and thinly sliced
- ½ large cucumber, seeds removed and sliced into half moons

1 In a large bowl, mix the herbs, lemon juice and zest and olive oil with some seasoning to make a dressing.
2 Add the butter beans, radishes and cucumber then mix the dressing through the salad.

Nutrition per serving
Kcals 209 • fat 5g • saturates 1g • carbs 27g • sugars 3g • fibre 13g • protein 13g • salt 0.6g

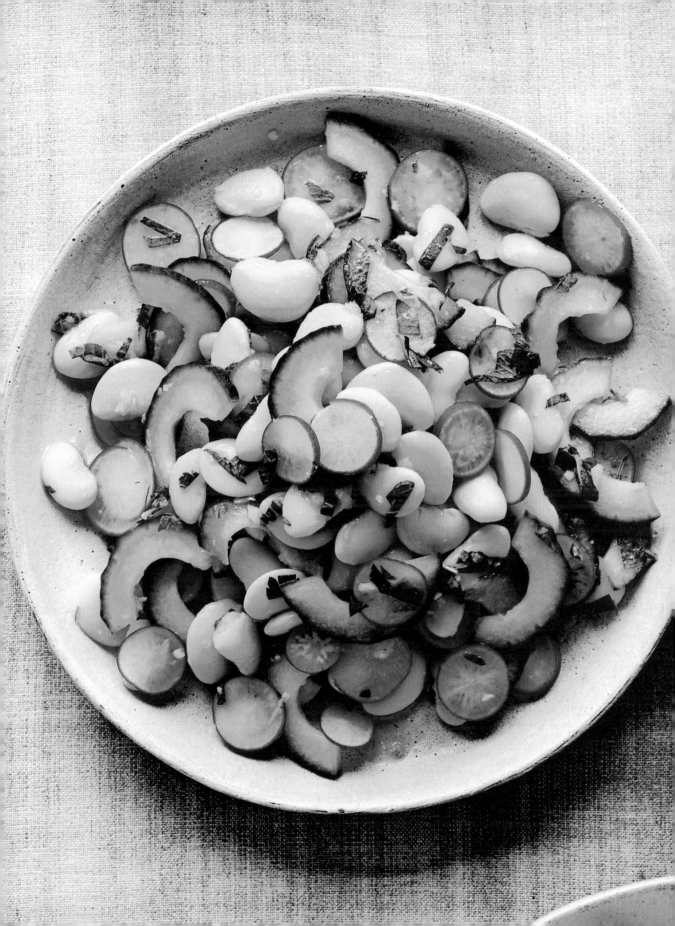

Herby potato salad

Try this potato salad at a barbecue for a different take on a classic summer salad. This delicious recipe instead features basil, parsley and garlic.

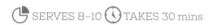 SERVES 8–10 TAKES 30 mins

- 1 large bunch basil
- 1 large bunch parsley
- 1kg new potatoes, larger potatoes halved
- 100ml extra virgin olive oil
- 2 tbsp white wine vinegar
- 1 small garlic clove

1 Bring a large pan of salted water to the boil, drop in the basil for 30 secs or until wilted, then fish out with a slotted spoon and set aside to cool slightly. Add the potatoes and cook until tender.

2 Meanwhile, squeeze out the basil over the sink, then put in a blender along with the oil, vinegar, garlic and a good pinch of seasoning. Blitz until you have a vibrant green oil.

3 Drain and steam-dry the potatoes. Chop the parsley, then tip it and the potatoes into a serving bowl. Season and toss in the basil oil. Will keep for 2 days.

Nutrition per serving (10)
Kcals 168 • fat 10g • saturates 2g • carbs 15g • sugars 1g • fibre 3g • protein 3g • salt 0.2g

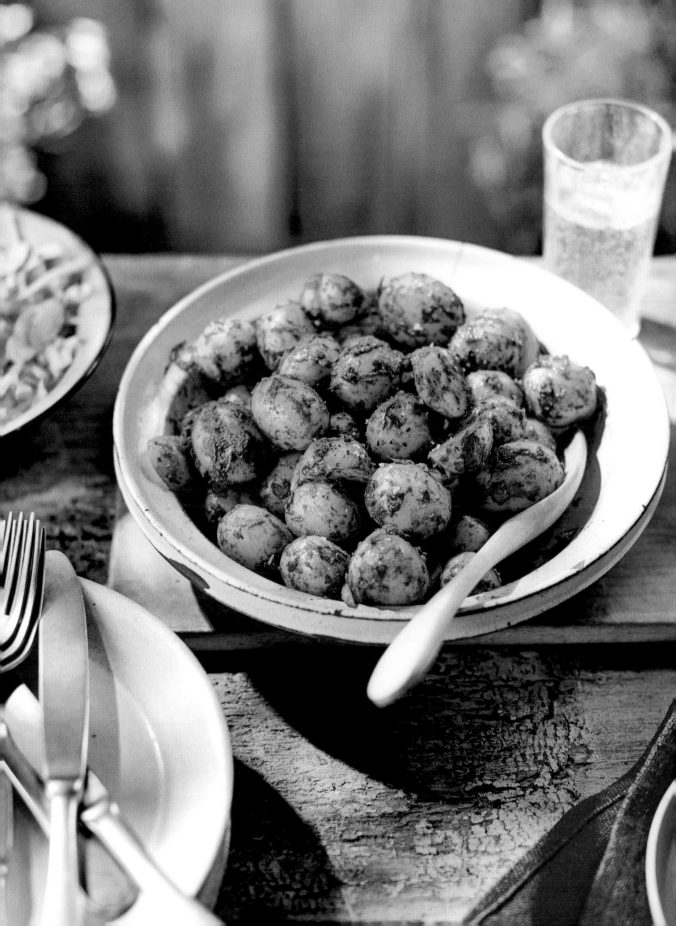

Grilled radicchio with fontina

Serve this grilled radicchio with fontina as a side dish or starter. If you can't find fontina cheese, parmesan or pecorino will be just as delicious.

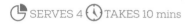 SERVES 4 TAKES 10 mins

- 2 radicchio heads, sliced through the core into wedges
- 2 tbsp olive oil, plus extra to serve
- 1 tbsp balsamic vinegar, plus extra to serve
- 2 tbsp thyme leaves
- 50g fontina, shaved or finely sliced

1 Heat grill to medium, around 160C. Lie the radicchio on a baking sheet and season. Whisk the oil and vinegar together, then drizzle over the radicchio. Grill for 5–8 mins, turning regularly – you want the veg to be softened and cooked through, but not too charred.
2 Serve on a large platter, topped with a scattering of thyme leaves and the fontina. Drizzle with a little more olive oil and balsamic vinegar, season, then serve.

Nutrition per serving
Kcals 145 • fat 10g • saturates 3g • carbs 7g • sugars 2g • fibre 2g • protein 6g • salt 0.4g

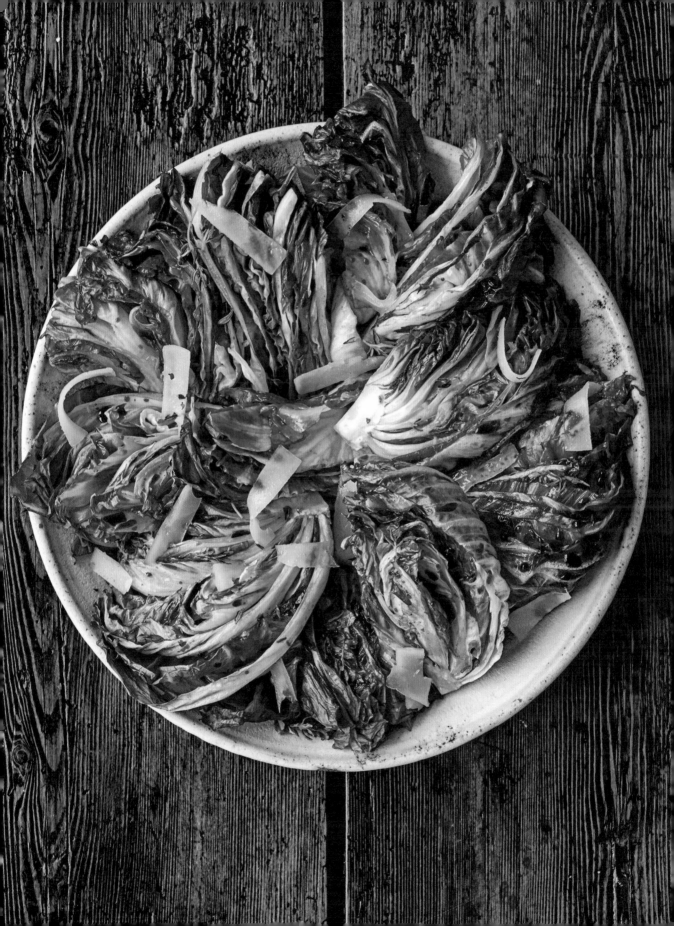

Best Yorkshire puddings

The secret to getting gloriously puffed-up Yorkshires is to have the fat sizzling hot and don't open the oven door!

MAKES 8 LARGE OR 24 SMALL · TAKES 30 mins

- sunflower oil, for cooking
- 140g plain flour (this is about 200ml)
- 4 eggs (200ml)
- 200ml milk

1 Heat oven to 230C/210C fan/gas 8. Drizzle a little sunflower oil evenly into 2 x 4-hole Yorkshire pudding tins or a 12-hole non-stick muffin tin and place in the oven to heat through.

2 To make the batter, tip the plain flour into a bowl and beat in the eggs until smooth. Gradually add the milk and carry on beating until the mix is completely lump-free. Season with salt and pepper. Pour the batter into a jug, then remove the hot tins from the oven. Carefully and evenly pour the batter into the holes. Place the tins back in the oven and leave undisturbed for 20–25 mins until the Yorkshire puddings have puffed up and browned. Serve immediately. You can now cool them and freeze for up to 1 month.

Nutrition per pud (8 large puds)
Kcals 199 · fat 13g · saturates 2g · carbs 15g · sugars 1g · fibre 0g · protein 6g · salt 0.12g

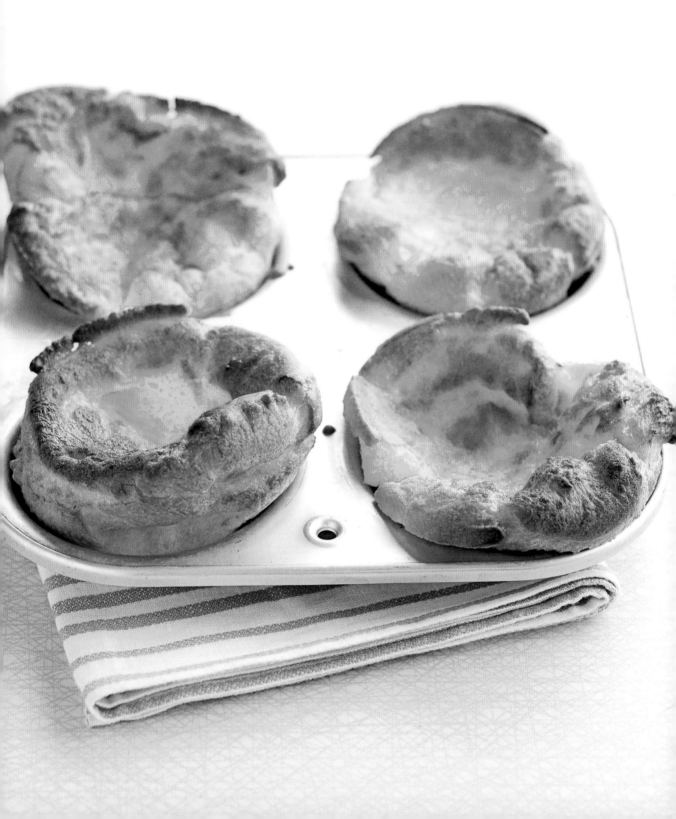

Best-ever oven chips

Make your own crispy, golden oven chips and save yourself some money. They're also much easier to cook than their fried counterparts.

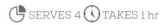 SERVES 4 TAKES 1 hr

- 1kg large Maris Piper potatoes, peeled
- 1 tbsp white or malt vinegar
- 75ml vegetable oil
- 2 tsp plain flour
- 2 tsp cornflour or potato flour
- ½ tsp baking powder

1 Trim all the rounded edges off the potatoes to make a rectangular block, then cut this into thick batons (save any offcuts to make mash). Drop into a pan of cold salted water with the vinegar and bring to the boil. Simmer for 6–8 mins until the potatoes are just cooked and tender – test with the tip of a knife. Drain carefully, trying not to break any of the chips, and leave to cool completely. Can be prepared up to 2 days ahead and chilled until needed.

2 Heat oven to 220C/200C fan/gas 7. Pour the oil into a sturdy, rimmed baking tray or shallow roasting tin and heat in the oven. Mix the flours with the baking powder and some salt in a shallow dish and gently toss the chips in the floury mixture to coat, then leave in the mixture until needed.

3 Carefully remove the pan from the oven – the oil should be shimmering – and lay the chips in a single layer in the pan. Use a thin, flexible spatula to gently turn the chips so they are all coated, then roast for 20 mins. Turn the chips again, then roast for another 10 mins. Turn one final time, then cook for a further 10 mins until crisp and deep golden all over. Drain the chips onto some kitchen paper and serve straight away.

OPTIONAL EXTRA
Try adding a pinch of cayenne pepper in with the flour for an extra kick.

Nutrition per serving
Kcals 409 • fat 19g • saturates 1g • carbs 53g • sugars 2g • fibre 4g • protein 4g • salt 0.5g

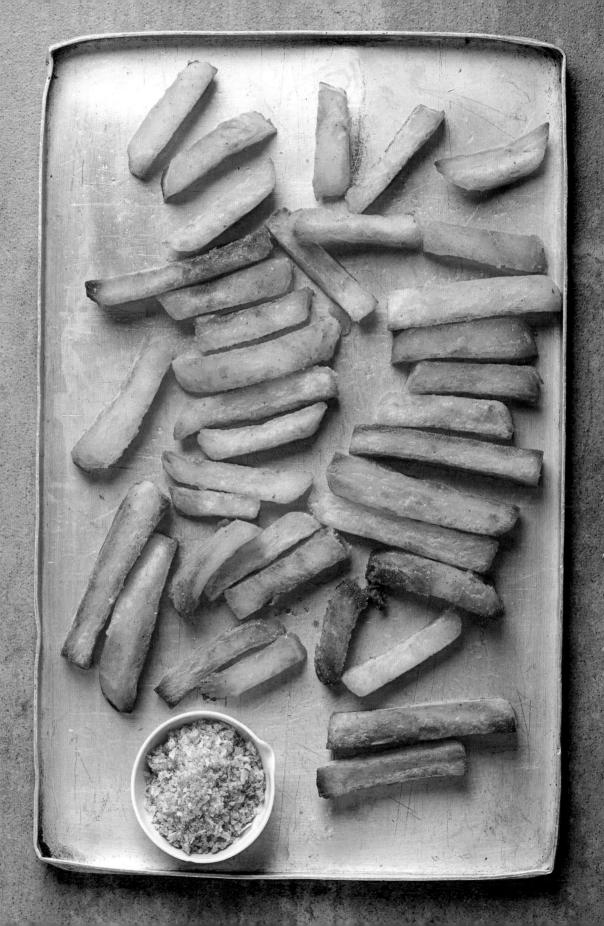

New potatoes with spinach and capers

Buttery new potatoes are a fantastic spring side to any dish. This zesty version with lemon, capers and greens offers a fresh and simple take.

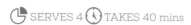 SERVES 4 TAKES 40 mins

- 500g new potatoes, halved
- 1 tbsp olive oil
- 2 tbsp butter
- 100g spinach
- 2 tbsp capers, drained and rinsed
- zest and juice ½ lemon

1 Put the potatoes in a large saucepan and cover with cold salted water. Bring to the boil, then simmer for 15 mins until they are tender but still hold their shape, and you can insert a cutlery knife easily.

2 Drain the potatoes and allow to steam-dry. Heat the oil with 1 tbsp of the butter in a large frying pan over a medium-high heat. Once the butter is foaming, add the potatoes, cut-side down, and fry undisturbed for 5 mins until golden.

3 Add the remaining butter along with the spinach, capers, lemon zest and juice. Stir everything together for a few mins so that the potatoes are coated and the spinach has wilted, then season to taste with salt and black pepper.

Nutrition per serving
Kcals 175 • fat 9g • saturates 4g • carbs 18g • sugars 2g • fibre 3g • protein 3g • salt 0.6g

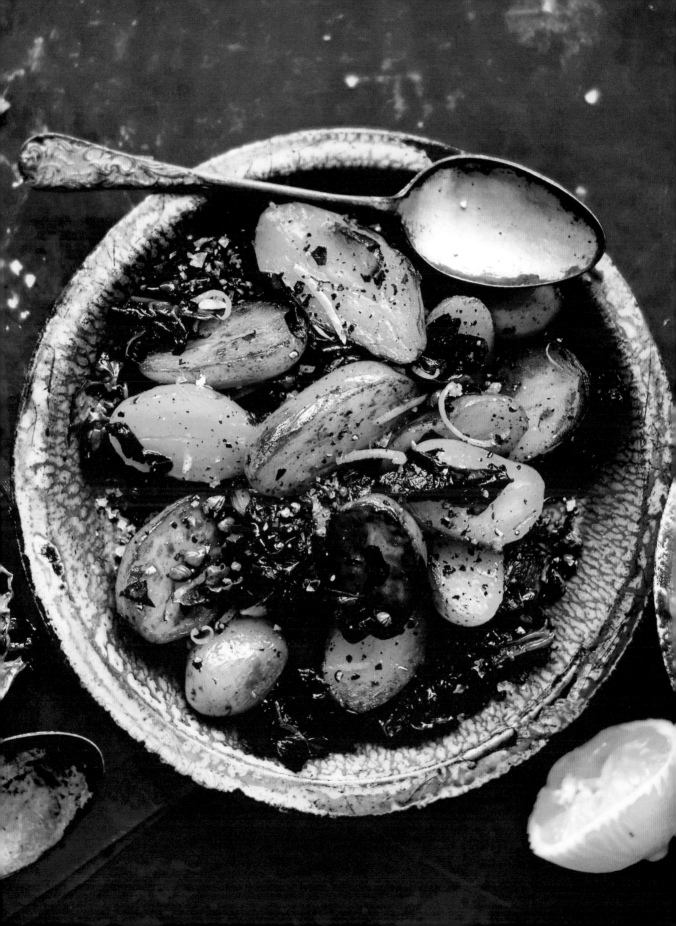

Sweet potato & chipotle mash

As an alternative to a classic comforting mash, try roasting sweet potatoes and crushing with spicy smoked chilli paste.

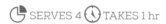 SERVES 4 TAKES 1 hr

- 4 large sweet potatoes, about 1kg
- 1 tbsp chipotle paste
- 125ml soured cream
- 25g butter

1 Heat oven to 200C/180C fan/gas 6. Put the potatoes in the oven and roast for 50 mins until tender when pierced with a knife. Peel off the skins, put the flesh in a bowl and mash until smooth.
2 Add the chipotle paste, soured cream and butter, and mix well. Season to taste.

Nutrition per serving
Kcals 330 • fat 12g • saturates 7g • carbs 51g • sugars 15g • fibre 8g • protein 4g • salt 0.5g

Herby buttermilk mash

This mash recipe involves beating your potatoes so the result is super-smooth. The mash is flavoured with parsley, dill and chives.

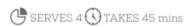 SERVES 4 TAKES 45 mins

- 900g Maris Piper potatoes, cut into chunks
- 50g butter
- 100ml buttermilk
- ½ tsp nutmeg, freshly grated
- 2 tbsp chopped mixed herbs (parsley, dill, chives)

1 Boil the potatoes in large pan of salted water, with the lid on, for 15–20 mins until tender. Drain well, return to the pan, cover and leave to steam-dry for 1–2 mins.
2 Remove from the heat and mash the potatoes until smooth. Push to one side of the pan, add the butter and buttermilk, then gently heat until the butter has melted. Beat in the potato a little at a time until smooth. Add the chopped herbs and season with ground white pepper and salt.

Nutrition per serving
Kcals 278 • fat 11g • saturates 7g • carbs 38g • sugars 3g • fibre 4g • protein 6g • salt 0.3g

Celeriac, cavolo nero & bacon mash

A new take on champ using Italian kale-like cabbage, bacon and celeriac, a versatile root that's lighter than potato.

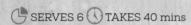 SERVES 6 ⏱ TAKES 40 mins

- 1½kg celeriac, peeled and cut into chunks
- 200g smoked bacon lardons
- 250g cavolo nero or green cabbage, finely shredded
- 50g butter
- 4 tbsp double cream

1 Boil the celeriac in a covered pan for 15–20 mins or until tender. Meanwhile, heat a frying pan and cook the bacon for 5 mins until golden and crisp. Add the cavolo nero or cabbage and cook over a low heat for 5 mins.

2 Drain the celeriac and blitz with a hand blender until smooth. Stir in the butter and cream. When the butter has melted, add the bacon and cavolo nero or cabbage, and stir well. Season to taste.

Nutrition per serving
Kcals 254 • fat 19g • saturates 10g • carbs 9g • sugars 5g • fibre 10g • protein 11g • salt 1.7g

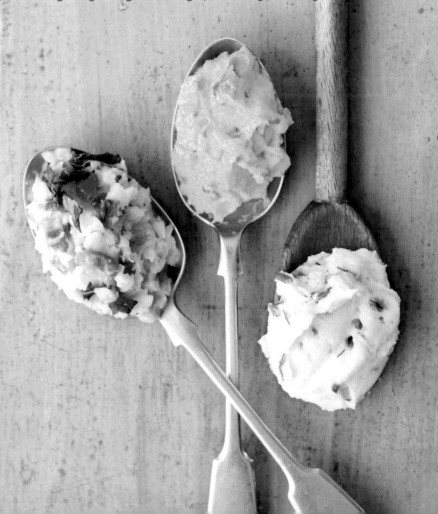

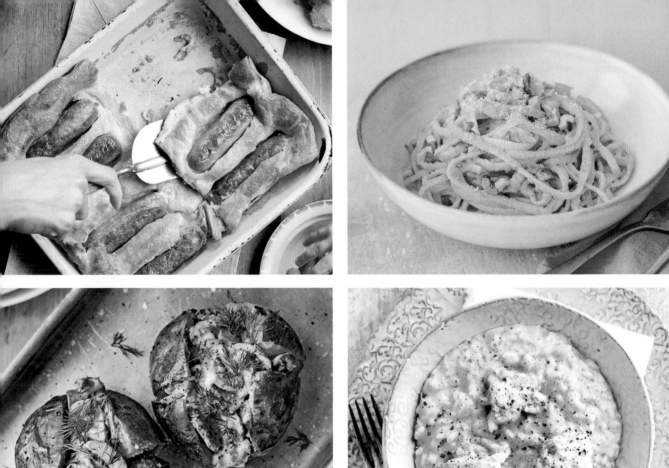

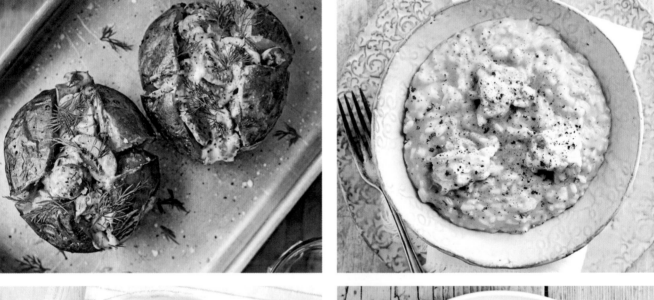

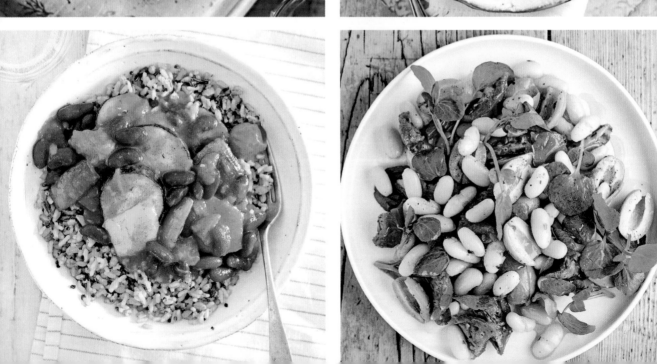

CHAPTER 4: VEGETARIAN MAINS

Vegetarian food needn't be reserved just for vegetarians, we'd all benefit from eating more vegetables. It's often cheaper than eating meat and the health benefits are multiple. And if you think vegetarian food is boring, think again. This chapter is full of exciting recipes that will give you a new-found love of veggies, grains and pulses. We've got pies, pasta, pizza and even toad-in-the-hole. Plenty of satisfying dinners, on the table with no fuss at all.

Sweet potato with red pepper halloumi

Top these barbecued sweet potatoes with red pepper and halloumi for a veggie alternative in a family summer feast. Serve with fresh herbs.

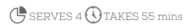 SERVES 4 TAKES 55 mins

- 4 medium sweet potatoes
- 1 tbsp olive oil
- small bunch parsley or mint, chopped
- 225g halloumi, cut into 4 slices
- 4 fat strips grilled red pepper
- 1 lemon, halved

1 Rub each potato with a little oil and salt, then wrap in a double layer of foil.
2 Pour the oil into a bowl and stir in half the herbs. Add the halloumi and toss until well coated in the oil. Wrap each piece in a strip of pepper. Cut 4 lengths of foil about 1cm wide and wrap one around the middle of each parcel to hold them together. You could use skewers instead, but be careful not to split the cheese.
3 Heat the barbecue. When the coals glow red, put the potatoes directly on them. Cook for 30 mins, turning halfway. Unwrap a potato and check if it is cooked through. If not, rewrap and cook more, checking every 10 mins. Alternatively, bake in the oven at 200C/180C fan/gas 6 for 50 mins–1 hr.
4 Meanwhile cook the pepper parcels on the barbecue or a griddle pan for 3–4 mins each side or until the pepper chars and the cheese melts a bit. Remove from the grill and unwind the foil or remove the skewers. Split the potatoes, then lay a parcel in the centre of each. Add a squeeze of lemon and scatter over some herbs to serve.

Nutrition per serving
Kcals 354 • fat 18g • saturates 11g • carbs 29g • sugars 16g • fibre 5g • protein 17g • salt 2g

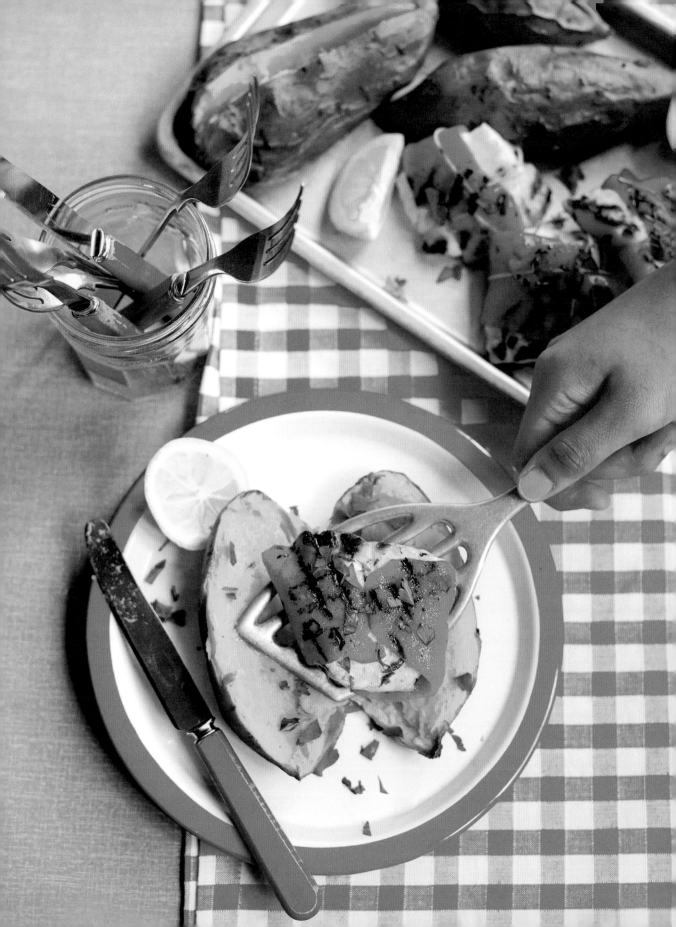

Squash quesadillas

Use just 4 ingredients to make our vegetarian quesdillas: butternut squash, feta, salad leaves and tortillas. Great for lunch or a quick midweek meal.

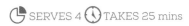 SERVES 4 TAKES 25 mins

- 350g chopped butternut squash
- 100g feta, crumbled
- 160g bag watercress, spinach & rocket
- 8 small flour tortillas
- olive oil, for drizzling

1 Heat oven to 200C/180C fan/gas 6. Boil the squash for 10 mins or until tender, drain and cool.
2 Divide the squash, feta and half the salad leaves over the tortillas and season well. Fold each tortilla into quarters, place on a baking tray and drizzle with a little olive oil. Put another baking tray on top and push down. Bake with the tray on top for 5 mins, then take the tray off and bake for a further 5 mins until golden. Serve with the remaining salad leaves.

Nutrition per serving
Kcals 362 • fat 12g • saturates 6g • carbs 48g • sugars 5g • fibre 5g • protein 13g • salt 1.9g

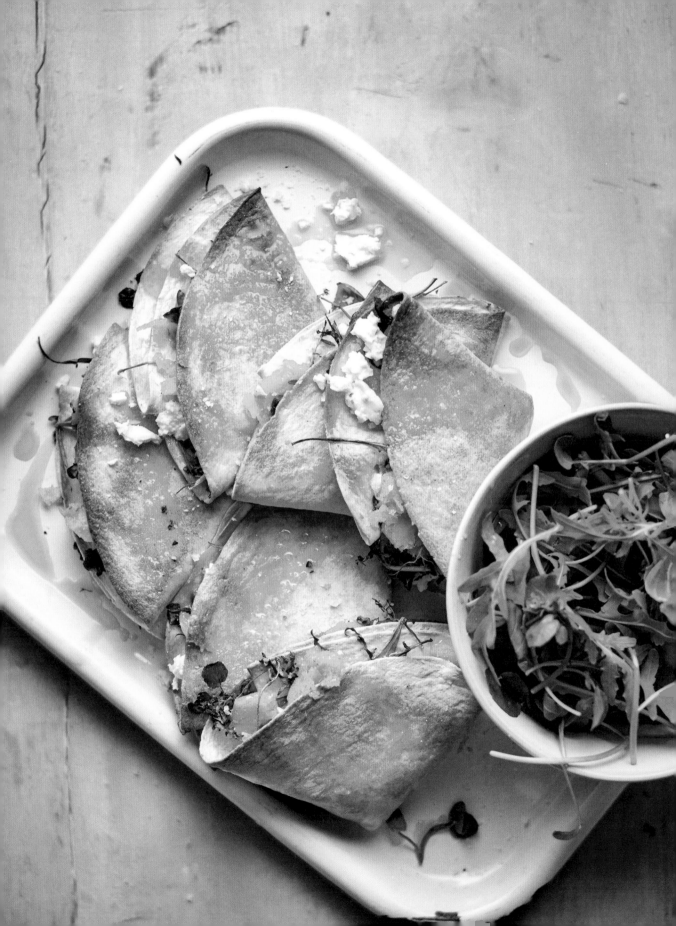

Veggie toad-in-the-hole

Use vegetarian sausages to make this moreish veggie toad-in-the-hole that's great for the whole family. Serve with vegetable side dishes and veggie gravy.

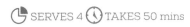 SERVES 4 TAKES 50 mins

- 2 tbsp rapeseed oil
- 8 vegetarian sausages

FOR THE BATTER
- 4 medium eggs
- 325ml semi-skimmed milk
- 250g plain flour

1 To make the batter, beat the eggs and milk together in a bowl, add 1 tsp salt, then beat again and leave to stand for 30 mins. Tip in the plain flour and beat well with a whisk until smooth. If you can, make this 2 hrs before needed and allow to stand before pouring into the tin.

2 Heat oven to 220C/200C fan/gas 7. Pour the oil in a 28 x 23cm roasting tin (or a tin roughly that size), coat the sausages in the oil and roast them in the oven for about 8–10 mins.

3 Stir the batter, then remove the tin from the oven and pour the batter over the hot oil and sausages (you can do this over a low heat on the hob to keep the oil nice and hot). Put the tin back in the oven and cook for 10 mins, then turn the temperature down to 180C/160C fan/gas 4 and cook for a further 25–30 mins or until the batter is golden and cooked through.

4 Test with a knife in the centre to check it's cooked. Serve with roast potatoes, carrots and veggie gravy, if you like, plus some green vegetables.

Nutrition per serving
Kcals 620 • fat 24g • saturates 4g • carbs 63g • sugars 7g • fibre 8g • protein 33g • salt 3.6g

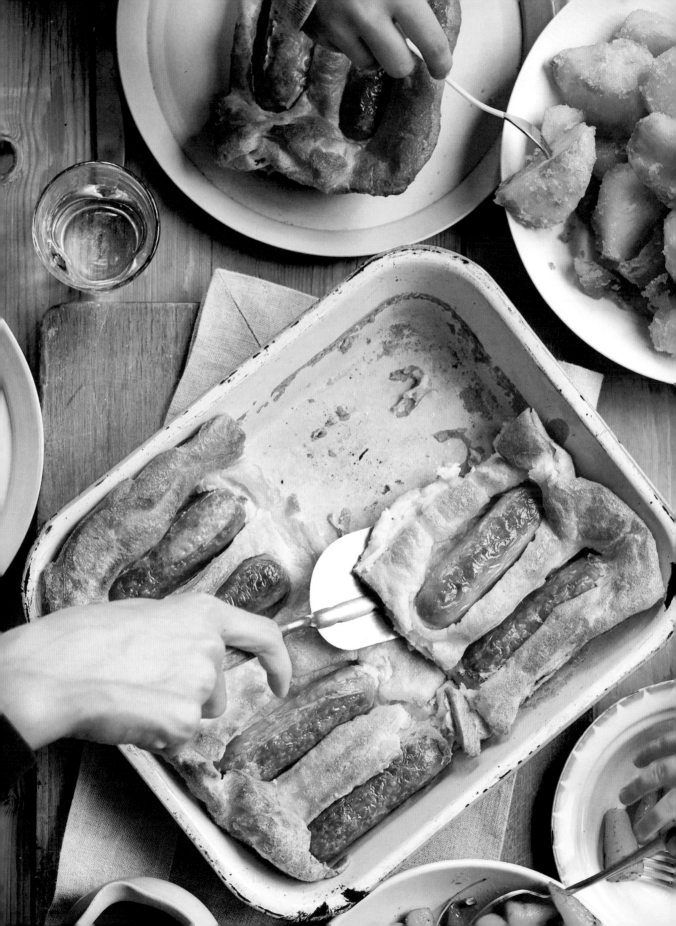

Crispy Greek-style pie

A crispy pie that you can adapt for your needs – add chicken or keep it veggie. A good fail-safe for your repertoire.

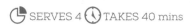 SERVES 4 TAKES 40 mins

- 200g bag spinach
- 175g jar sundried tomatoes in oil
- 100g feta cheese, crumbled
- 2 eggs
- ½ 250g pack filo pastry

1 Put the spinach into a large pan. Pour over a couple tbsp water, then cook until just wilted. Tip into a sieve, leave to cool a little, then squeeze out any excess water and roughly chop. Roughly chop the tomatoes and put into a bowl along with the spinach, feta and eggs. Mix well.

2 Carefully unroll the filo pastry. Cover with some damp sheets of kitchen paper to stop it drying out. Take a sheet of pastry and brush liberally with some of the sundried tomato oil. Drape oil-side down in a 22cm loose-bottomed cake tin so that some of the pastry hangs over the side. Brush oil on another piece of pastry and place in the tin, just a little further round. Keep placing the pastry pieces in the tin until you have roughly 3 layers, then spoon over the filling. Pull the sides into the middle, scrunch up and make sure the filling is covered. Brush with a little more oil.

3 Heat oven to 180C/fan 160C/gas 4. Cook the pie for 30 mins until the pastry is crisp and golden brown. Remove from the cake tin, slice into wedges and serve with salad.

Nutrition per serving
Kcals 250 • fat 13g • saturates 5g • carbs 23g • sugars 5g • fibre 3g • protein 13g • salt 0.3g

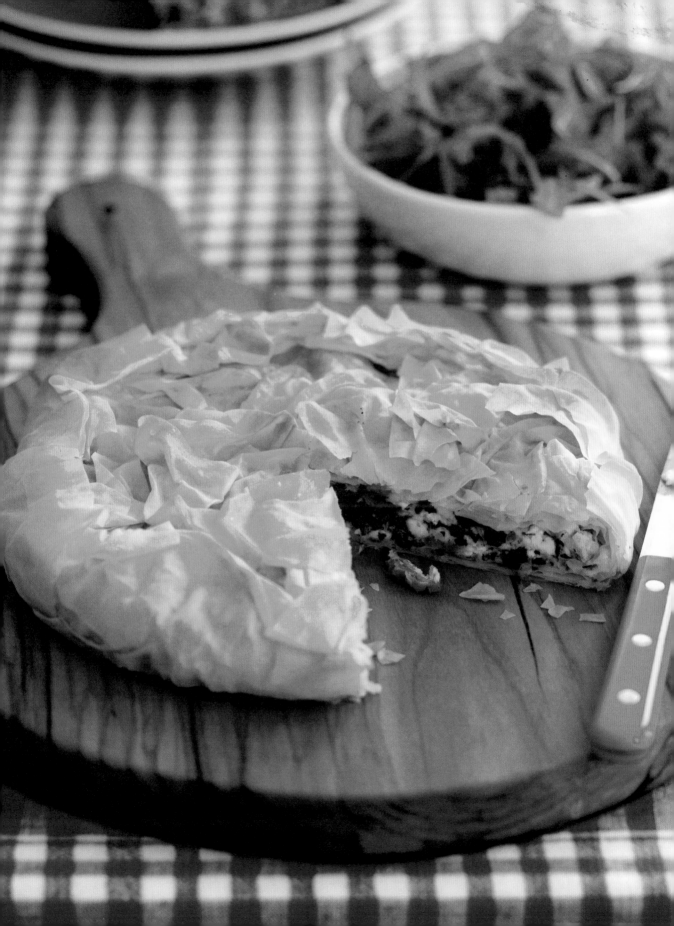

Cheat's aubergine parmigiana

A cheat's way to create that classic Italian dish, aubergine parmigiana, with just 4 ingredients and no fuss. Assemble this family-friendly meal in minutes.

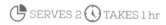 SERVES 2 TAKES 1 hr

- 2 medium aubergines
- 2 tbsp olive oil
- 400g can chopped tomatoes
- 2 x 125g balls buffalo mozzarella
- 30g grated parmesan (or vegetarian alternative)

1 Heat oven to 200C/180C fan/gas 6. Put the aubergines on a baking tray and make a slit down the centre of each. Drizzle with olive oil and season. Bake for 50–55 mins or until the flesh is soft. Heat the grill. Tip the tomatoes into a bowl and season well. Fill the aubergines with layers of tomatoes and mozzarella, and finish with the parmesan. Put under the grill for 5–7 mins until the cheese is golden.

Nutrition per serving
Kcals 596 • fat 42g • saturates 22g • carbs 15g • sugars 14g • fibre 11g • protein 33g • salt 1.5g

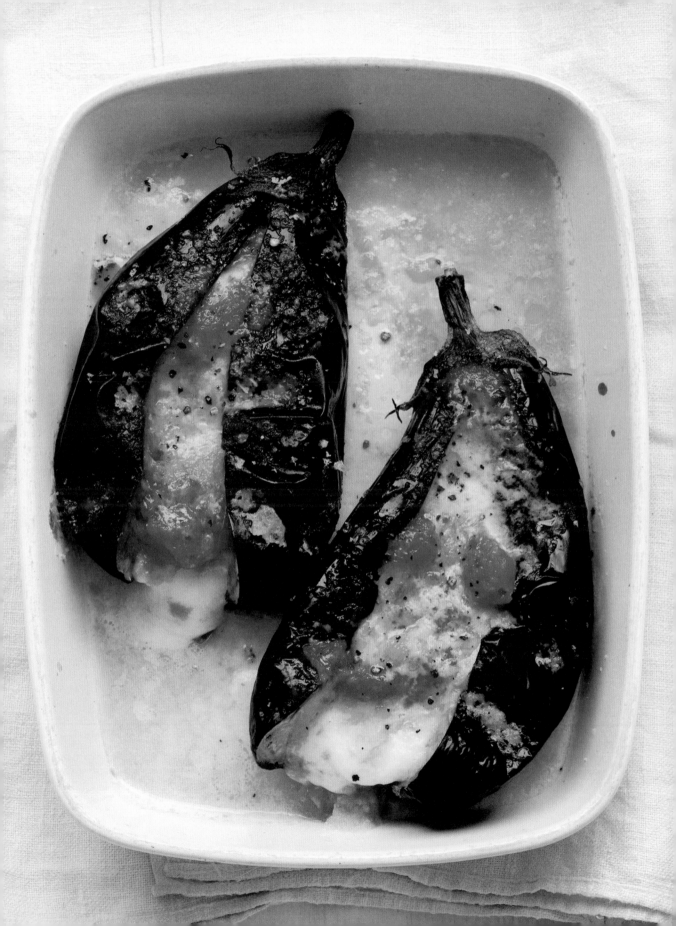

Spinach & halloumi salad

Try this tasty spinach and halloumi salad as a light main or starter. It contains just 4 ingredients so is super simple to make, and it's super speedy too.

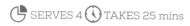 SERVES 4 ⏱ TAKES 25 mins

- 250g halloumi cheese
- 200g bag spinach
- 1 bunch mint, leaves only
- 2 large oranges
- 2 tbsp olive oil

1 Slice the halloumi and griddle for 3–4 mins each side until charred, then set aside. Tip the spinach and half the mint onto a large platter. Segment the oranges and pour any orange juice from the chopping board into a bowl, and squeeze the pith to get juices from there too. Scatter the orange pieces over the spinach. Chop the remaining mint and mix with the orange juice, olive oil and some seasoning. Place the halloumi slices on top of the salad and pour the dressing over. Serve with warm flatbreads.

Nutrition per serving
Kcals 297 • fat 21g • saturates 11g • carbs 10g • sugars 9g • fibre 2g • protein 17g • salt 1.9g

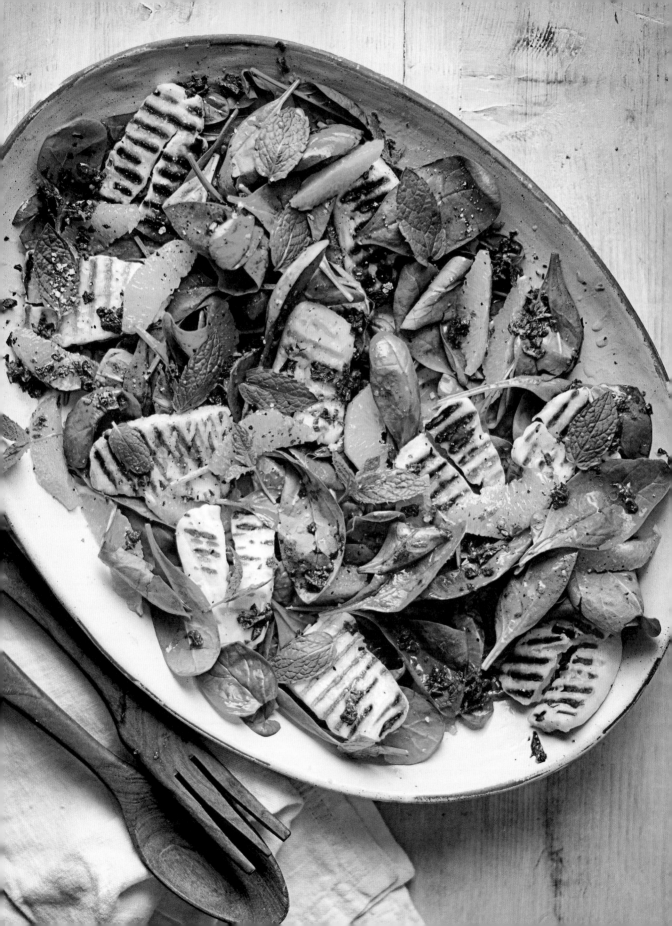

Roasted feta

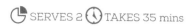

Try this simple way to cook with feta. Using just 4 ingredients – feta, veg antipasti, lemon and pitta bread – you can serve up a delicious lunch for 2.

SERVES 2   TAKES 35 mins

- 2 x 185g packs chargrilled veg antipasti
- 1 lemon
- 200g vegetarian feta
- olive oil, for drizzling
- 2 large wholemeal pittas

1 Heat oven to 180C/160C fan/gas 4. Tip the antipasti and its oil into a roasting tin, squeeze over the lemon juice, reserving the zest, and place the feta in the middle of the tin. Season with black pepper and drizzle over a little extra olive oil. Bake in the oven for 25 mins. Toast the pittas for 1–2 mins until warmed through. Scatter the lemon zest over the feta. Serve with the pittas.

Nutrition per serving
Kcals 540 • fat 28g • saturates 15g • carbs 40g • sugars 15g • fibre 10g • protein 26g • salt 7.9g

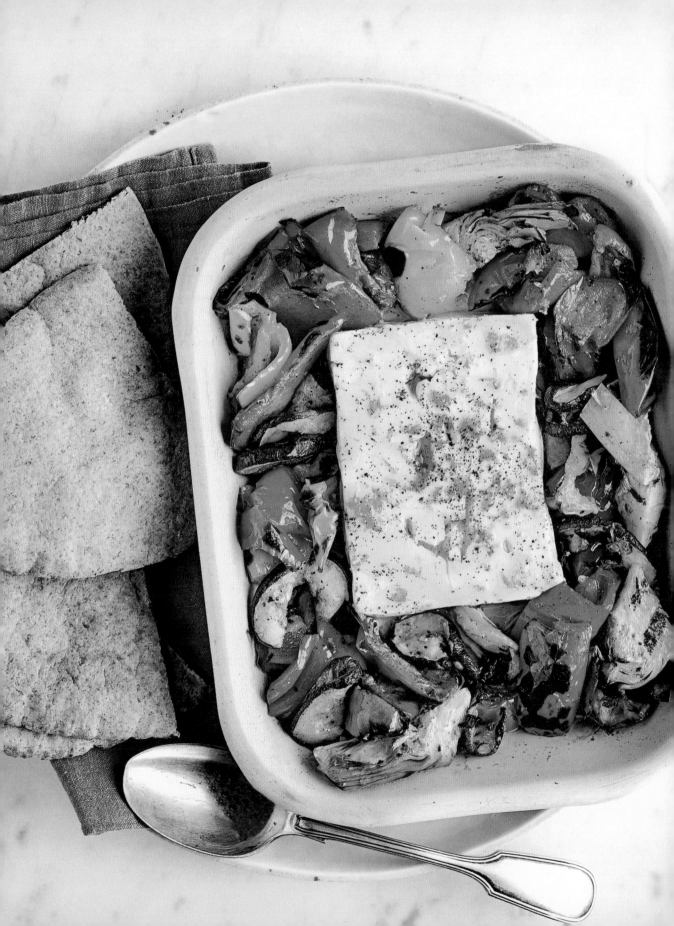

Vegetarian chilli

The easiest chilli you'll ever make, with ready-to-eat grains, kidney beans in chilli sauce and summer veggies – it's 4 of your 5-a-day too!

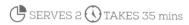 SERVES 2 TAKES 35 mins

- 400g pack oven-roasted vegetables
- 400g can kidney beans in chilli sauce
- 400g can chopped tomatoes
- 1 ready-to-eat mixed grain pouch

1 Heat oven to 200C/180C fan/ gas 6. Cook the vegetables in a casserole dish for 15 mins. Tip in the beans and tomatoes, season, and cook for another 10–15 mins until piping hot. Heat the pouch in the microwave on High for 1 min and serve with the chilli.

Nutrition per serving
Kcals 608 • fat 14g • saturates 2g • carbs 88g • sugars 30g • fibre 21g • protein 22g • salt 2.4g

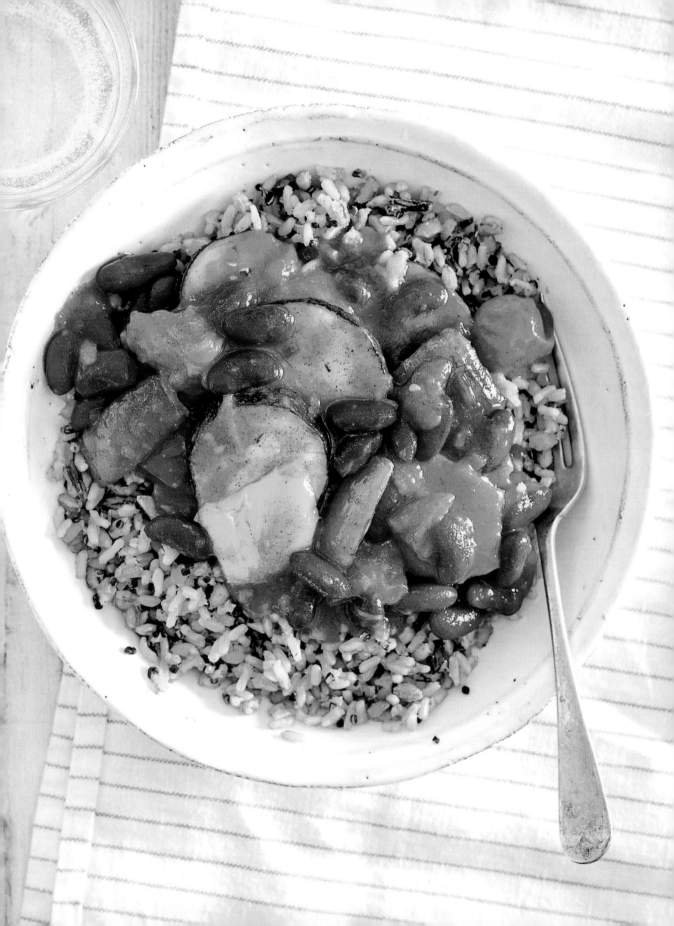

Squash & lentil salad

Make this butternut squash and lentil salad for a low-calorie, gluten-free lunch or dinner, or as a side dish. It's easy to make, with just a few ingredients.

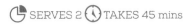 SERVES 2 TAKES 45 mins

- 350g chopped butternut squash
- 4 tbsp olive oil
- 75g cucumber & mint raita or tzatziki
- 250g pouch Puy lentils
- small bunch dill

1 Heat oven to 220C/200C fan/gas 7. Toss the squash in 2 tbsp olive oil, season and roast for 30–35 mins or until golden.
2 Add 2–3 tsp water to the raita, stir until smooth and set aside. Toss the lentils with half the raita, squash and dill. Tip the lentils onto a plate, top with remaining squash, drizzle over the remaining olive oil and the rest of the raita. Garnish with the remaining dill.

Nutrition per serving
Kcals 409 • fat 19g • saturates 4g • carbs 39g • sugars 9g • fibre 11g • protein 16g • salt 1.6g

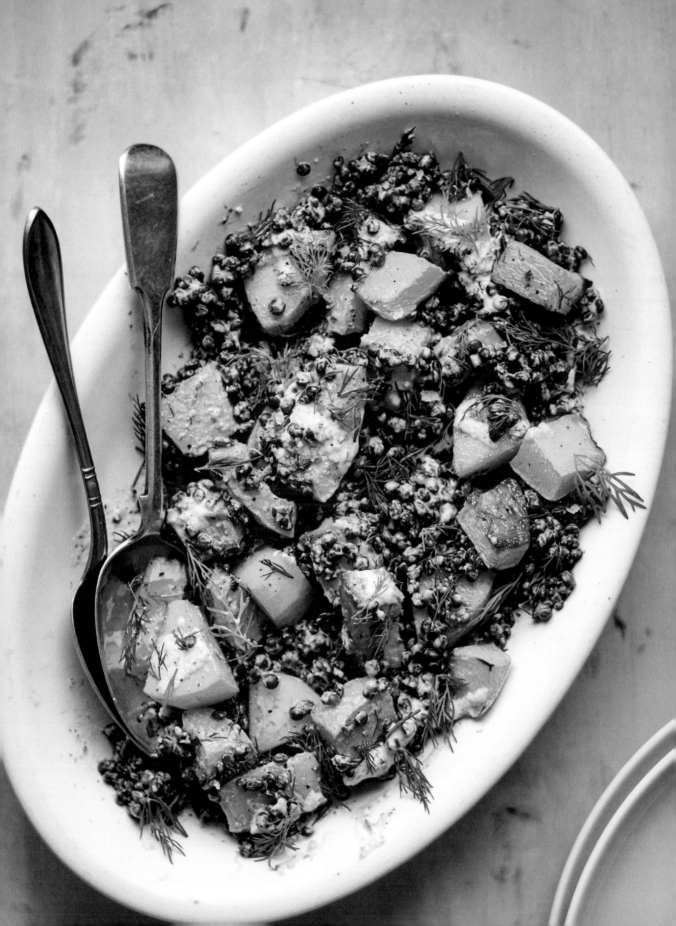

Bean, tomato & watercress salad

Try this gluten-free, vegan salad with filling beans and fresh watercress for a quick, light meal. It has just 4 ingredients and 3 of your 5-a-day.

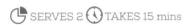 SERVES 2 TAKES 15 mins

- 2 x 400g cans cannellini beans
- 100g watercress
- zest and juice 1 lemon
- 250g pack sundried tomatoes and olives

1 Drain and rinse the beans, then combine in a bowl with the watercress, zest and juice of the lemon, tomatoes and olives, including the oil from the pack. Toss well and season to taste.

Nutrition per serving
Kcals 454 • fat 23g • saturates 3g • carbs 40g • sugars 5g • fibre 10g • protein 16g • salt 4.8g

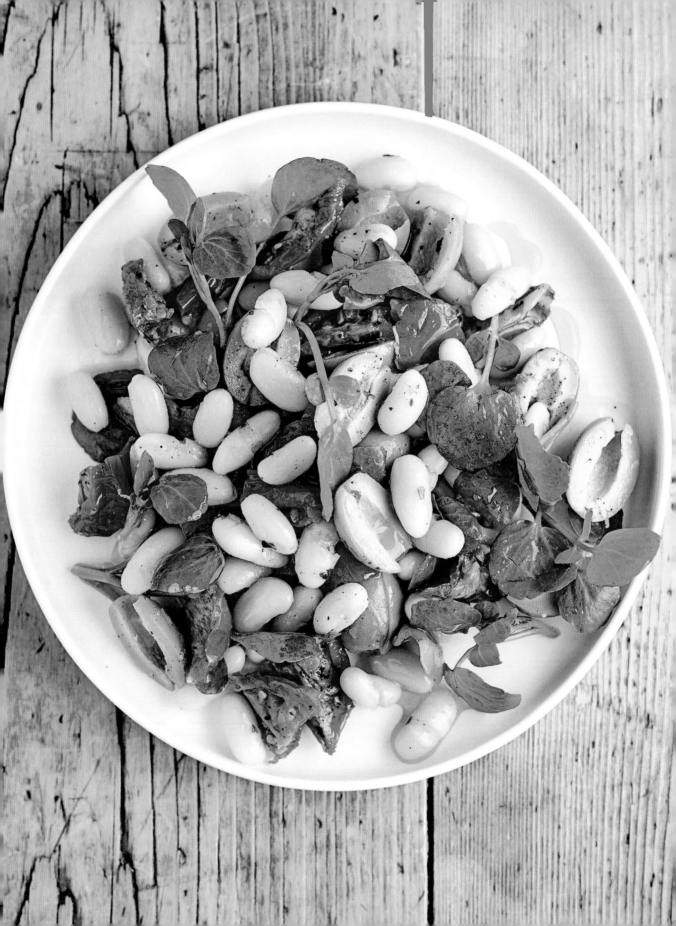

Cheat's gnudi

Transform a bag of spinach with this cheat's gnudi – gnocchi-like dumplings made with cheese instead of potato. You only need 4 ingredients and 25 minutes.

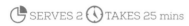 SERVES 2 TAKES 25 mins

- 200g bag spinach
- 150g garlic & herb Boursin
- 100g fresh breadcrumbs
- oil, for drizzling
- 2 tbsp grated parmesan (or vegetarian alternative)

1 Put the spinach in a large colander set over the sink. Pour boiling water over, then leave to cool and drain. Squeeze out the excess moisture, then blitz in a food processor with the soft cheese, breadcrumbs and some seasoning. Rub some oil on your hands, then shape the mixture into 20 balls. Cook in a pan of boiling, salted water for 2 mins. Scoop out, season and drizzle over some oil and scatter over the parmesan.

Nutrition per serving
Kcals 502 • fat 36g • saturates 23g • carbs 24g • sugars 3g • fibre 2g • protein 19g • salt 1.8g

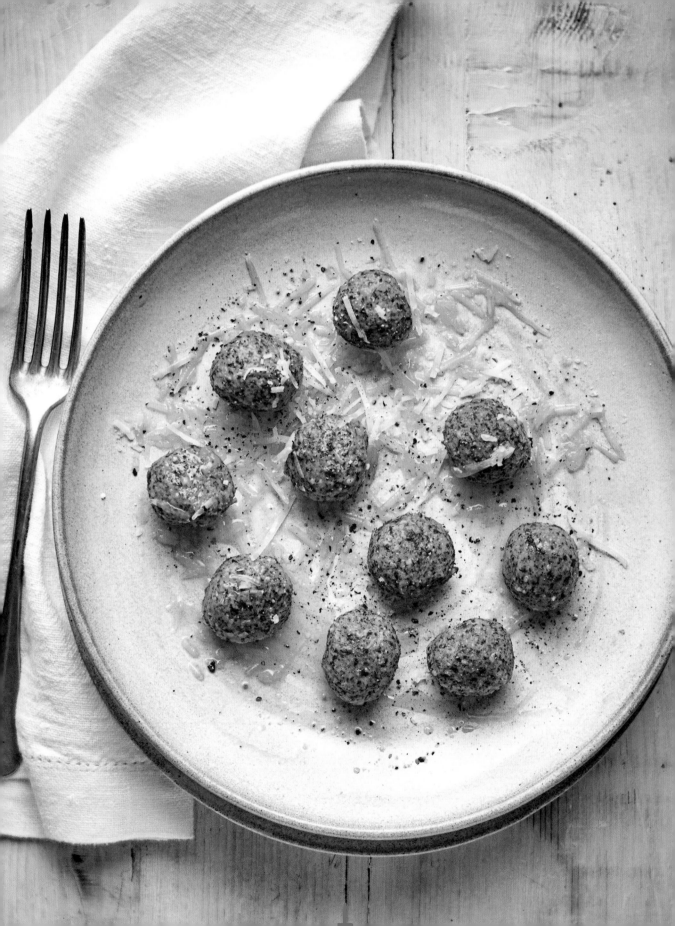

Creamy squash linguine

Rustle up this healthy pasta dish using just a handful of ingredients.

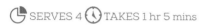 SERVES 4 ⏱ TAKES 1 hr 5 mins

- 350g chopped butternut squash
- 3 tbsp olive oil
- 4 garlic cloves, skins on
- 350g linguine
- small bunch sage
- parmesan (or vegetarian alternative), to serve (optional)

1 Heat oven to 200C/180C fan/gas 6. Put the squash on a baking tray, drizzle with the olive oil and season well. Roast for 25 mins. Add the garlic and cook for another 10–15 mins until soft.

2 Cook the pasta according to pack instructions. Drain, reserving the water. Squeeze the garlic cloves from their skins, use a stick blender to whizz with the squash with 400ml cooking water, taste it and add extra seasoning if you need to. Heat some oil in a frying pan, fry the sage until crisp, then drain on kitchen paper. Tip the pasta and sauce into the warm oil in the pan and heat through. Scatter with sage and parmesan, if you like.

Nutrition per serving
Kcals 441 • fat 11g • saturates 2g • carbs 71g • sugars 5g • fibre 6g • protein 12g • salt 0g

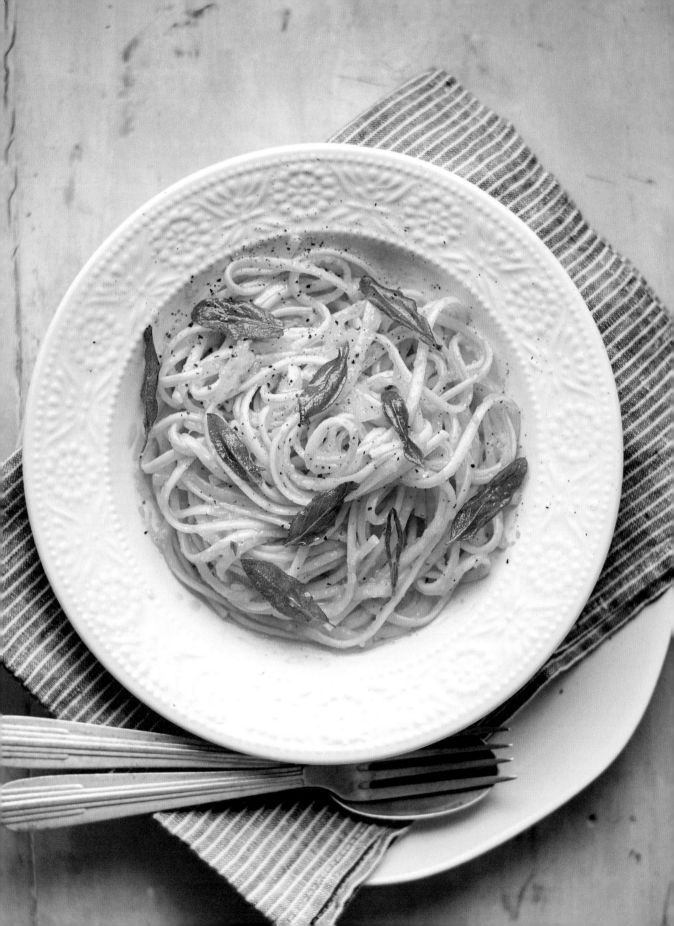

Beetroot, hummus & chickpea sub sandwich

Load up a sub with homemade hummus, beetroot, chickpeas and salad to make this filling vegan sandwich. An ideal lunch for when hunger strikes.

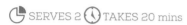 SERVES 2 TAKES 20 mins

- 300g pack cooked beetroot in water, drained, half sliced
- 400g can chickpeas, drained
- 3 tbsp vegetarian pesto
- olive oil
- 2 large ciabatta rolls, sliced in half
- 2 large handfuls mixed rocket, watercress & spinach salad

1 Blitz the whole beetroot, ¾ of the chickpeas, 2 tbsp pesto and 1 tbsp oil in a food processor with some seasoning until you have a thick, smooth hummus. Heat the ciabatta following the pack instructions.
2 Fry the remaining chickpeas in a little oil until crisp, then set aside. Toss the salad leaves with the remaining pesto. Slice the rolls, then assemble the sandwiches with the hummus, beetroot slices, salad leaves and fried chickpeas.

Nutrition per serving
Kcals 639 • fat 22g • saturates 3g • carbs 77g • sugars 16g • fibre 14g • protein 24g • salt 1.6g

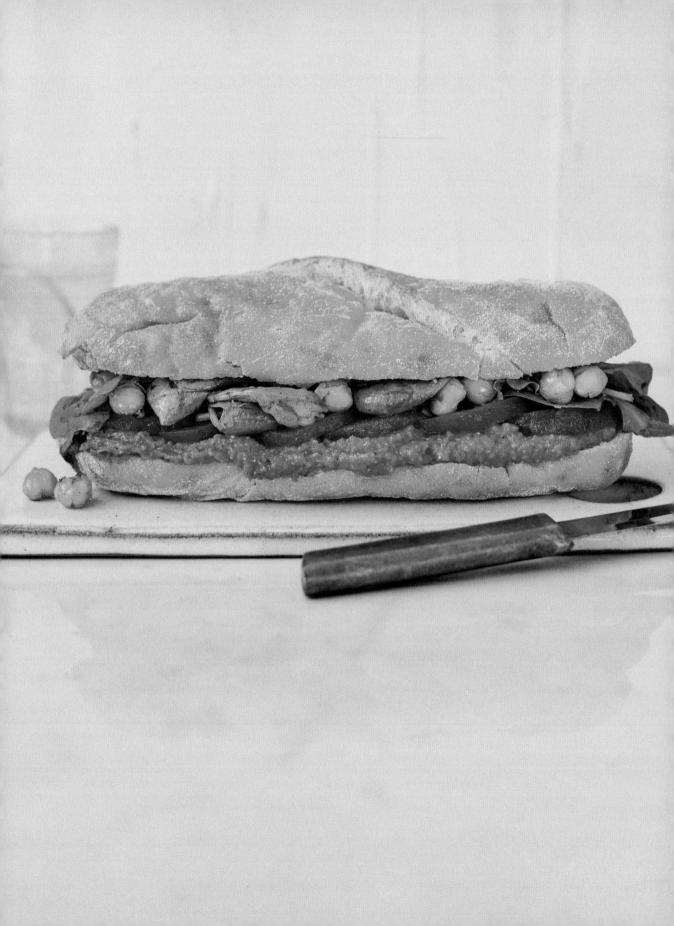

Artichoke & watercress linguine

Whip up this tasty vegetarian linguine dish in 25 minutes with just 4 ingredients. Full of flavour, it also contains 2 of your 5-a-day.

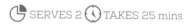 SERVES 2 ⏱ TAKES 25 mins

- 100g watercress
- 280g jar artichokes in olive oil
- 60g ricotta
- 220g linguine

1 Blitz together the watercress, ¾ of the artichokes, the ricotta and 3 tbsp olive oil from the jar, then season to taste.
2 Bring a large pan of salted water to the boil and cook the linguine following pack instructions until al dente. Toss the pasta with the watercress pesto along with the remaining artichokes and a ladleful of pasta water. Finish with an extra drizzle of olive oil and black pepper.

Nutrition per serving
Kcals 679 • fat 27g • saturates 5g • carbs 84g • sugars 3g • fibre 13g • protein 19g • salt 2.3g

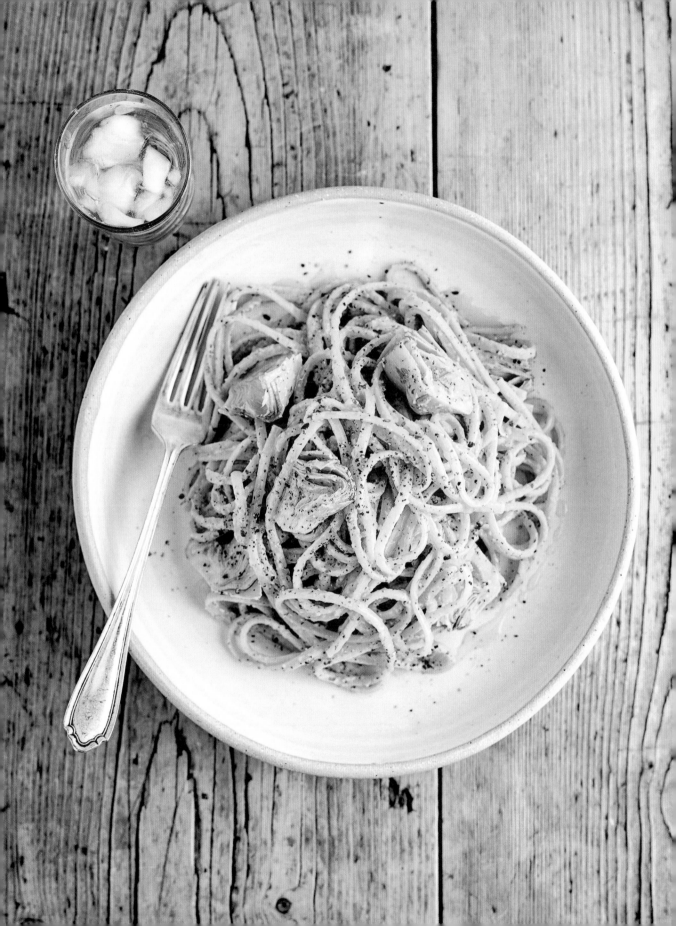

Spinach & chickpea dhal

Make this quick and easy dhal with just 4 ingredients: chickpeas, spinach, coconut cream and aubergine pickle. It's vegan, gluten-free and so tasty.

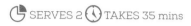 SERVES 2 ⓘ TAKES 35 mins

- 400g can chickpeas
- 1 tbsp sunflower oil
- 200g bag spinach
- 1 tbsp curry paste, we used balti
- 160ml can coconut cream
- 1 tbsp aubergine pickle

1 Heat oven to 220C/200C fan/gas 7. Drain the chickpeas, reserving the liquid, then tip ½ of them onto a baking tray, season, drizzle over 2 tsp sunflower oil and roast for 15 mins.

2 Wilt the spinach in a frying pan with 1 tsp sunflower oil and the curry paste, then add the coconut cream, remaining chickpeas and pickle. Mix well and simmer for 3–4 mins, squashing the chickpeas with the back of a spoon. Add a splash of the chickpea liquid if it looks dry. Sprinkle the roasted chickpeas on top and serve with naan bread.

Nutrition per serving
Kcals 522 • fat 38g • saturates 25g • carbs 26g • sugars 7g • fibre 8g • protein 15g • salt 0.4g

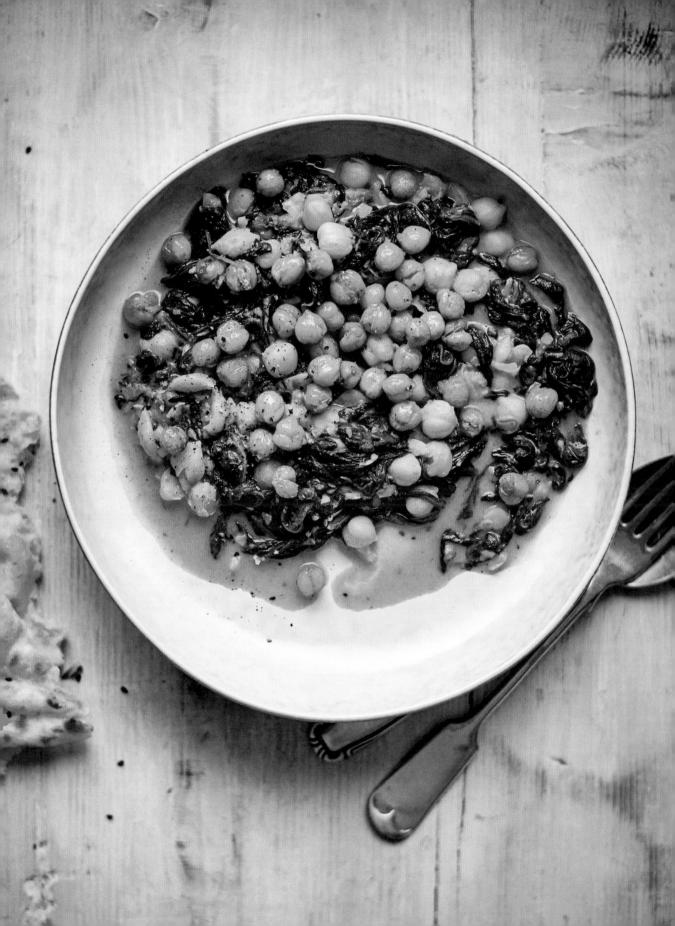

Mushroom jacket potatoes

Take just a few ingredients and rustle up these tasty mushroom jacket potatoes. They're healthy, low-calorie, gluten-free and ideal for a filling lunch or supper.

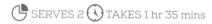 SERVES 2 TAKES 1 hr 35 mins

- 2 large potatoes
- 2 tsp sunflower oil
- 250g mushrooms
- 100g sour cream and chive dip
- sprigs of dill (to garnish)

1 Heat oven to 200C/180C fan/gas 6. Prick the potatoes all over with a fork and rub with half the sunflower oil. Bake the potatoes for 1 hr 20 mins.

2 Slice the mushrooms, fry in the remaining oil, then stir through half the sour cream and chive dip. Pile the mushrooms into the jacket potatoes and garnish with dill.

Nutrition per serving
Kcals 383 • fat 14g • saturates 4g • carbs 51g • sugars 4g • fibre 7g • protein 10g • salt 0.3g

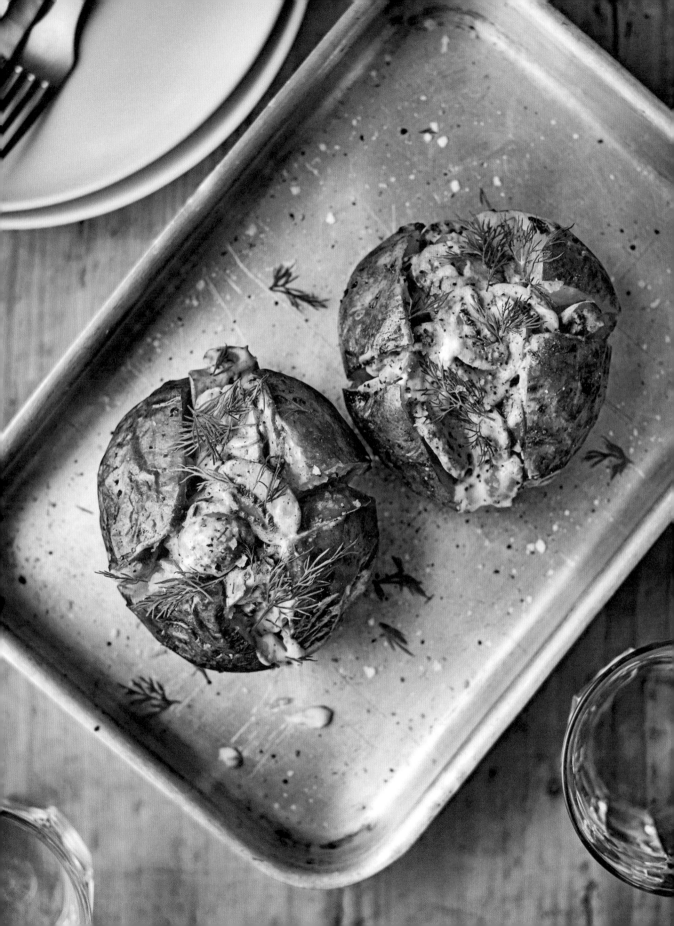

Baked polenta with spinach & goat's cheese

Try a new way to use polenta in this Italian inspired bake.

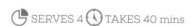 SERVES 4 TAKES 40 mins

- 3 garlic cloves, chopped
- 2 x 400g cans chopped tomatoes
- 300g fresh spinach
- 500g pack ready-made polenta
- 1 tbsp olive oil
- 100g goat's cheese with rind, broken into chunks

1 Heat oven to 220C/200C fan/gas 7 and boil the kettle. In a bowl, mix the garlic and tomatoes with seasoning, then pour into a large baking dish. Place the spinach in a large colander and pour boiling water over until wilted. Rinse in cold water and squeeze out all the excess water you can with your hands. Roughly chop, season, and scatter on top of the tomatoes.

2 Slice the polenta, then overlap on top of the spinach. Drizzle with the oil and bake in the oven for 10–15 mins. Scatter over the cheese and return to the oven for 5 mins more, or until the cheese is golden and bubbling.

Nutrition per serving
Kcals 240 • fat 10g • saturates 5g • carbs 26g • sugars 7g • fibre 6g • protein 12g • salt 1.6g

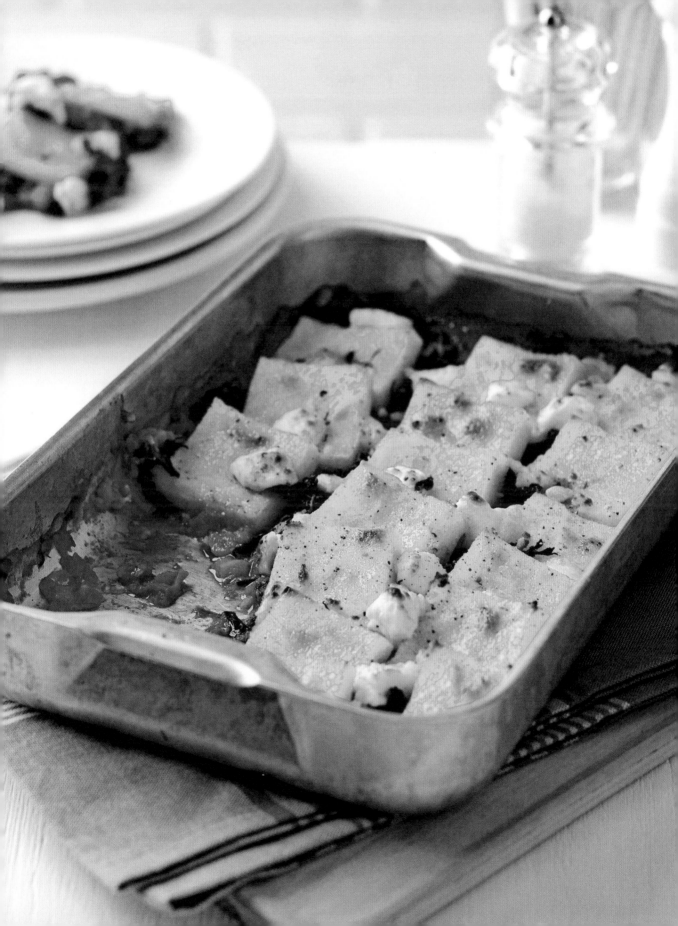

Red pepper linguine

Dig out a red pepper, linguine, walnuts, garlic and parmesan to make this quick and easy supper. It takes just 20 minutes from prep to plate.

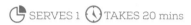 SERVES 1 TAKES 20 mins

- 1 roasted red pepper (from a jar or roast one yourself)
- 30ml olive oil
- 50g walnuts, toasted, plus extra to serve
- 1 small garlic clove
- 100g linguine or spaghetti
- parmesan (or vegetarian alternative), grated, to serve

1 Blitz the roasted red pepper with the olive oil, walnuts and garlic in a food processor, season well and set aside.

2 Bring a pan of salted water to the boil, add the pasta and cook for 1 min less than the pack instructions and drain, reserving a ladleful of cooking water. Tip the pasta back into the pan, along with the reserved cooking water and red pepper sauce, and return to the heat to warm through. Tip the pasta into a bowl and top with the parmesan and some chopped toasted walnuts. Season and serve.

Nutrition per serving
Kcals 1011 • fat 66g • saturates 8g • carbs 78g • sugars 3g • fibre 7g • protein 23g • salt 0.2g

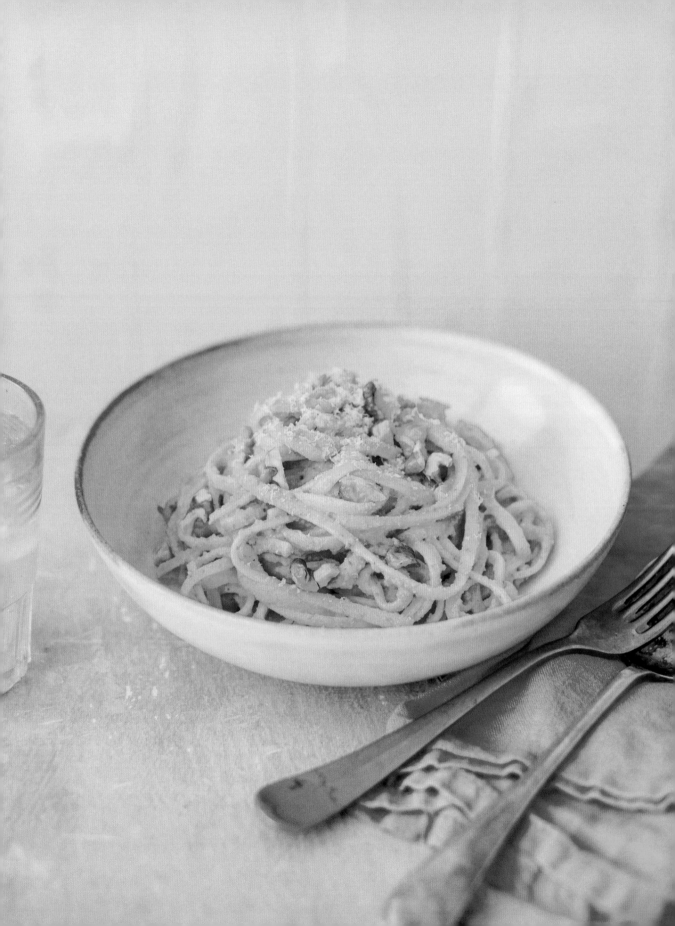

Asparagus cream pasta

Making a cream out of the stalks means that every mouthful of pasta will have a delicious taste of asparagus.

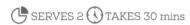 SERVES 2 TAKES 30 mins

- 1 bunch asparagus
- 142ml tub double cream
- 2 garlic cloves, peeled, but left whole
- 50g parmesan (or vegetarian alternative), half grated, half shaved
- 250g tagliatelle

1 To prepare the asparagus, cut off and discard the woody ends, then neatly cut the tips away from the stalks. Keep the tips and stalks separate. In a small saucepan bring the cream and garlic to the boil. Take off the heat, remove the garlic, then set the pan aside.

2 Cook the stalks in boiling salted water for about 4–5 mins until tender, drain, then tip into the cream with the grated parmesan. Blitz with a hand blender until smooth.

3 Cook the pasta according to pack instructions, then throw in the tips 2 mins before the end of cooking time. Gently reheat the cream, drain pasta, then tip into a bowl with the cream. Toss, divide into pasta bowls, top with parmesan shavings and serve.

Nutrition per serving
Kcals 931 • fat 47g • saturates 26g • carbs 100g • sugars 5g • fibre 5g • protein 28g • salt 0.53g

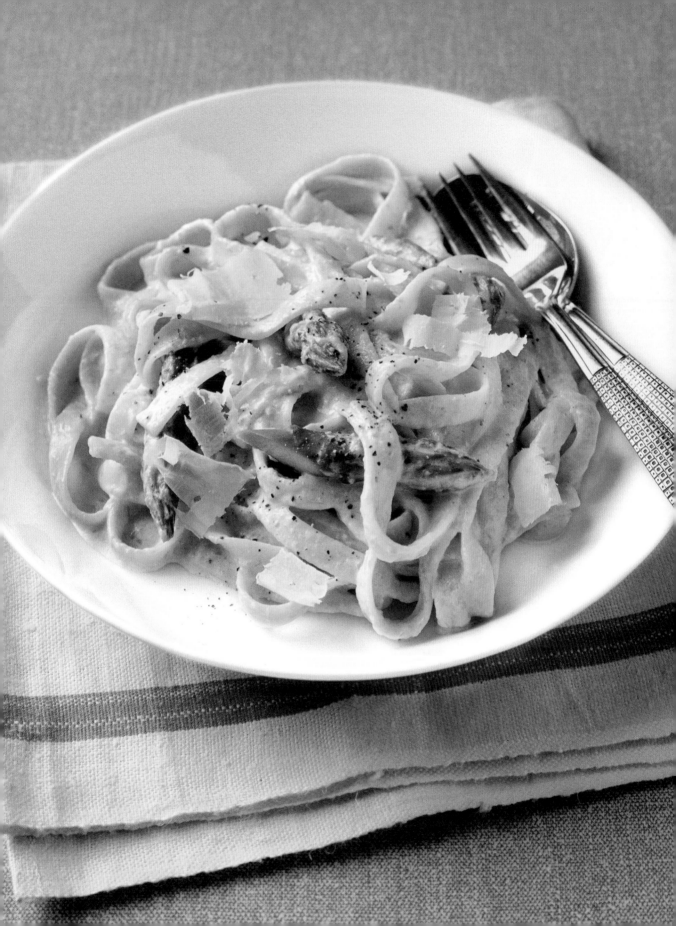

Next level Margherita pizza

Forget takeaways – you can't beat a homemade Margherita pizza topped with fresh tomato sauce and melted cheese. Here's how to master this everyday classic …

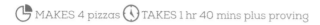 MAKES 4 pizzas ⏱ TAKES 1 hr 40 mins plus proving

- 300g jar tomato pasta or pizza sauce

FOR THE DOUGH
- 500g '00' or strong white flour, plus extra for dusting
- 1 sachet (7g) fast-action dried yeast

FOR THE TOPPINGS
- 50g parmesan (or vegetarian alternative), freshly grated
- 200g mozzarella from a block, cut into chunks
- olive oil, for drizzling

1 First, make the dough. Tip the flour into a bowl and add 300ml tepid water. Mix together and set aside at room temperature for 1 hr. Dissolve the yeast in 2 tbsp water and mix this and 15g of salt through the dough. Cover with cling film and leave somewhere warm to double in size for a few hours. For a sourer flavour, leave in the fridge for at least 8 hrs and up to 24 hrs – the longer you leave it the sourer it will be.
2 When the dough is ready, tip it onto a lightly floured surface and divide into 4. Roll into balls and leave to rest, covered with a tea towel or cling film, for another hour.
3 To make the pizza, heat a grill to its highest setting and get a heavy frying pan. On a floured surface push and stretch one of the balls of dough out into a circle roughly the same size as the frying pan. Slip the round onto a floured baking sheet and top with a quarter of the sauce, a scattering of parmesan and a quarter of the mozzarella.
4 Get the pan very hot and carefully slide the pizza onto it. Cook for 2 mins, then put the pan under the grill for another 2 mins until the sides are puffed up and the cheese has melted. Lift onto a board, drizzle with a little olive oil if you like, then cut into wedges and serve while you make the next one.

Nutrition per serving
Kcals 693 • fat 18g • saturates 10g • carbs 98g • sugars 4g • fibre 5g • protein 31g • salt 4.5g

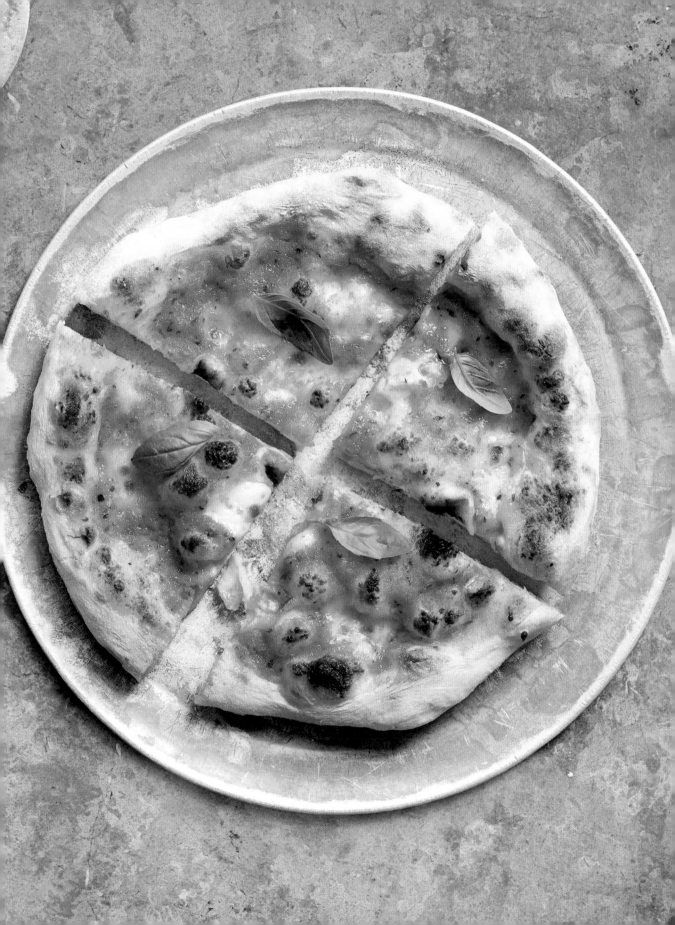

Creamy tomato courgetti

A quick low-calorie supper, ready in just 5 minutes. Swap the courgette for pasta if you want something more substantial.

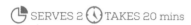 SERVES 2 TAKES 20 mins

- 4 slices prosciutto
- 200g can chopped tomatoes
- 100g mascarpone
- 250g pack courgetti
- ½ small pack basil, leaves picked

1 Heat a frying pan over a medium heat and dry-fry the prosciutto until crisp. Transfer to a plate with a slotted spoon. Add the tomatoes to the pan and bubble for 10 mins with some seasoning, until they thicken to a sauce. Stir in the mascarpone and bubble for another minute. Toss the courgetti through the sauce. Cook for 1 min more until warmed through. Divide between bowls, then top with the ham and basil.

Nutrition per serving
Kcals 300 • fat 19g • saturates 9g • carbs 15g • sugars 9g • fibre 2g • protein 16g • salt 3.1g

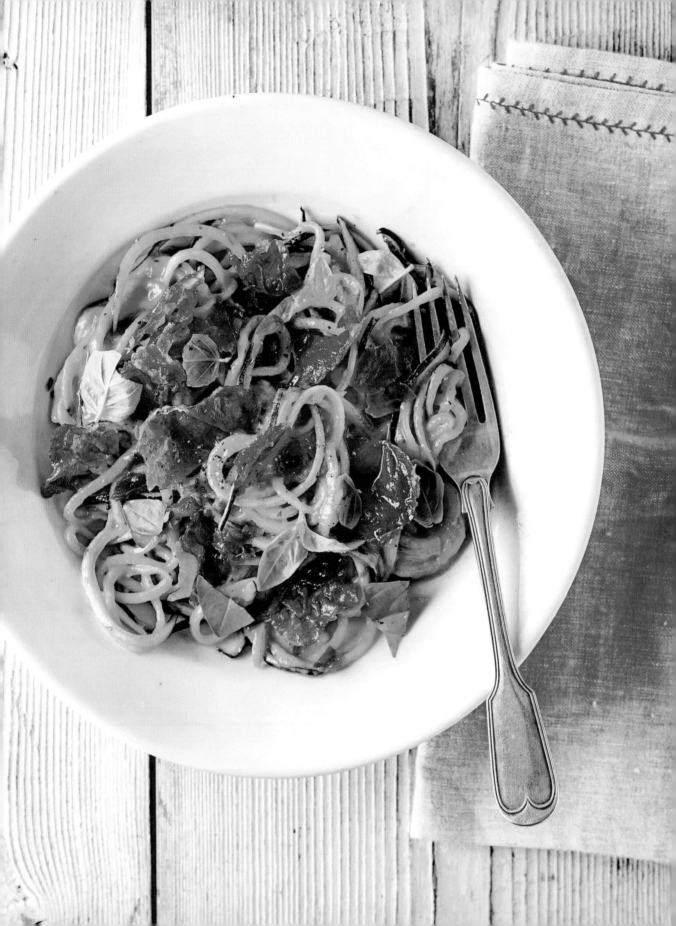

Pesto & goat's cheese risotto

A risotto that's bursting with fresh Italian flavours – simple to make, it's the perfect no-fuss midweek meal for 2.

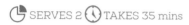 SERVES 2 TAKES 35 mins

- olive oil, for frying
- 200g risotto rice
- 700ml chicken stock or vegetable stock
- 1 tub fresh pesto
- 100g soft goat's cheese

1 Pour a glug of olive oil into a large saucepan. Tip in the rice and fry for 1 min. Add half the stock and cook until absorbed. Add the remaining stock, a ladle at a time, and cook until the rice is al dente, stirring continually, for 20–25 mins.

2 Stir through the pesto and half the goat's cheese. Serve topped with the remaining cheese.

Nutrition per serving
Kcals 745 • fat 32g • saturates 12g • carbs 83g • sugars 2g • fibre 4g • protein 29g • salt 2.4g

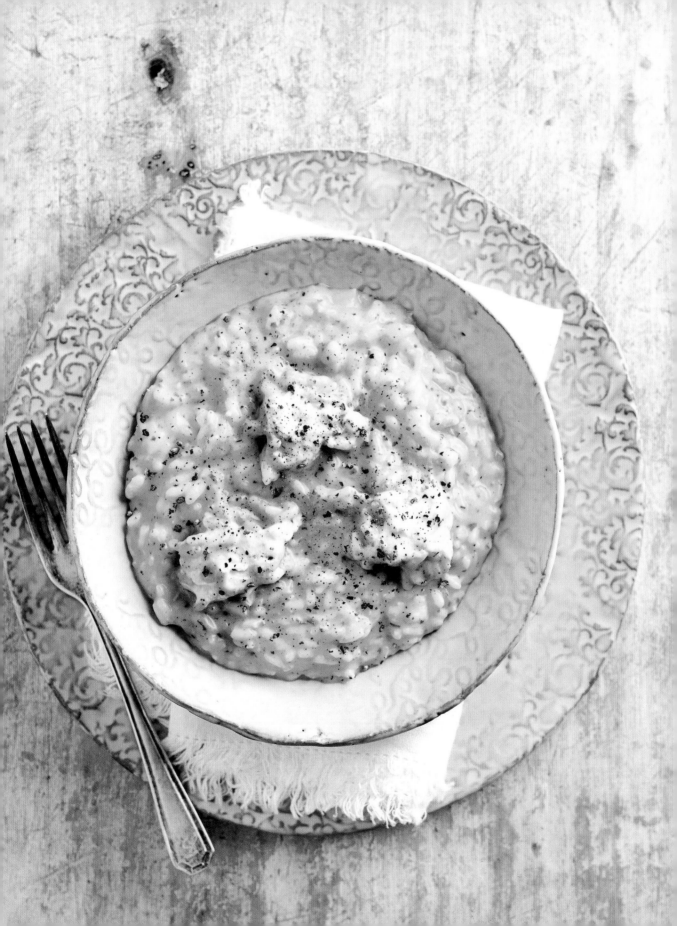

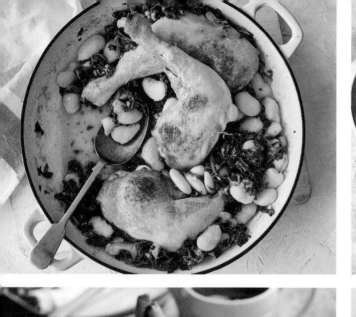

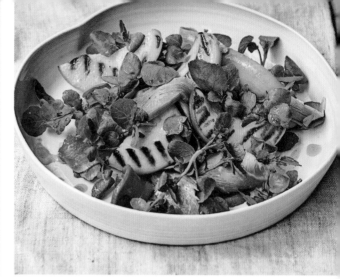

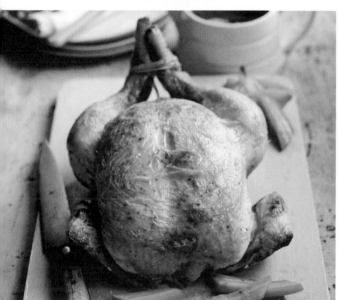

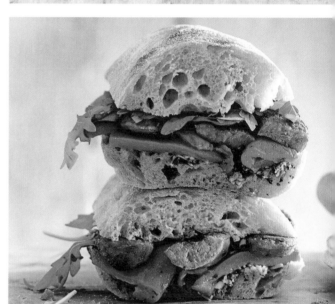

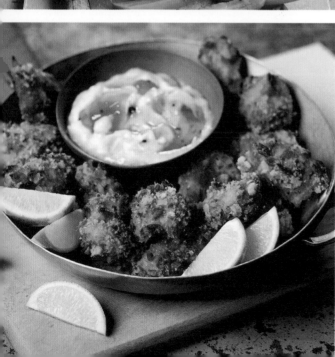

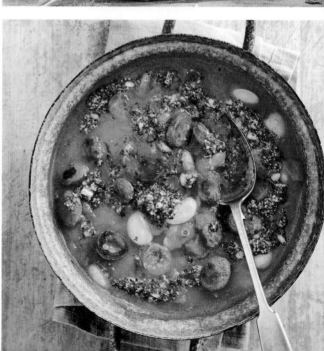

CHAPTER 5: MEAT & POULTRY

Whether you're looking for a quick dinner for the kids or something fancy to impress friends, you'll find everything you need in this chapter. We've included recipes for a variety of different meats and poultry, and with chicken being the most popular meat in the UK, there's plenty of inspiration for it in here. If your kids love chicken nuggets, try our spicy tikka version for something a bit different. The Smoked duck & peach salad is simple and perfect for entertaining, and the carbonara is not to be missed.

BBQ chicken & blue cheese wedges

A quick and easy midweek meal that kids and adults will love. If you don't like blue cheese you can replace it with cheddar.

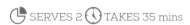 SERVES 2 ⟐ TAKES 35 mins

- 2 sweet potatoes (400g)
- 1 tbsp oil
- 2 chicken breasts
- 5 tbsp barbecue sauce
- 75g Stilton

1 Scrub the sweet potatoes and cut each into 6 wedges. Spread out on a baking sheet, drizzle with the oil, season and roast at 200C/180C fan/gas 6 for 20 mins.
2 Lightly bash the breasts between 2 pieces of cling film until about 1cm thick. Put the chicken in a bowl and coat in the BBQ sauce. Add the chicken to the baking sheet, return to the oven for 10 mins, then crumble the cheese over the potatoes and bake for 5 mins more until bubbling.

Nutrition per serving
Kcals 579 • fat 21g • saturates 10g • carbs 53g • sugars 22g • fibre 7g • protein 41g • salt 1.7g

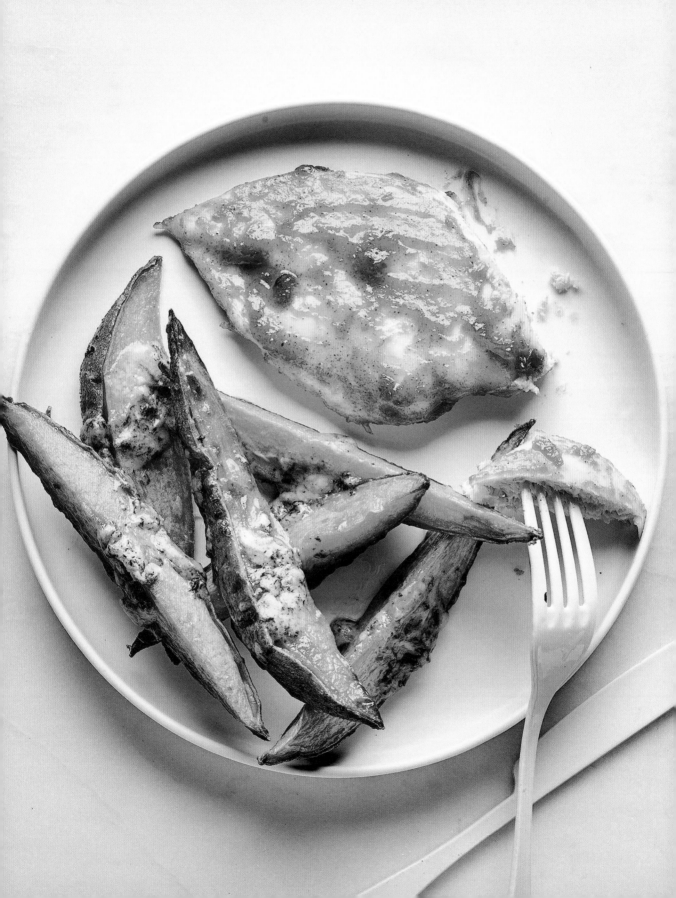

Crispy prosciutto chicken

This simple, filling chicken supper is low calorie and full to the brim with fibre.

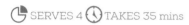 SERVES 4 TAKES 35 mins

- 8 skinless boneless chicken thighs
- 8 slices prosciutto
- 2 x 250g pouches Puy lentils
- 280g jar sundried tomatoes
- 1½ tbsp red wine vinegar

1 Heat oven to 180C/160C fan/gas 4. Wrap each chicken thigh in 1 slice of prosciutto and place on a baking tray. Drizzle with olive oil, season and bake for 30 mins until crispy and cooked through. Meanwhile, put the lentils in a medium saucepan and gently warm through with the sundried tomatoes, half their oil and the vinegar. Spoon the warm lentils onto 4 plates and top with the chicken.

Nutrition per serving
Kcals 467 • fat 10g • saturates 3g • carbs 41g • sugars 15g • fibre 13g • protein 47g • salt 3.4g

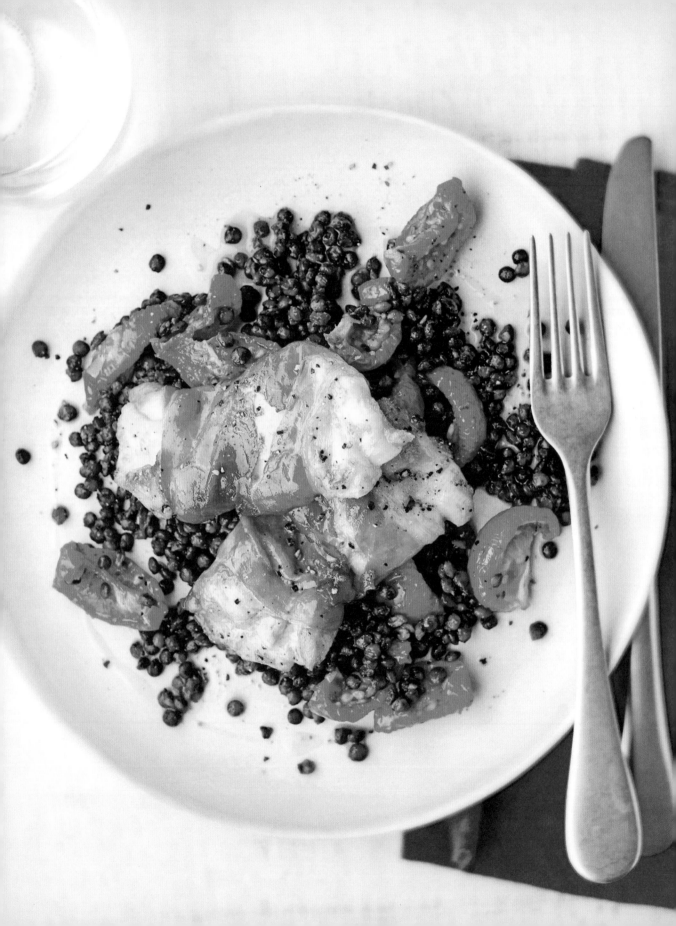

Chicken tikka nuggets

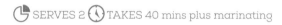

Give chicken nuggets a modern makeover with our tikka spices and mango chutney dip. Serve as party nibbles with mayo and lime – they won't last long.

SERVES 2 TAKES 40 mins plus marinating

- 500g chicken thighs
- 150ml natural yogurt, plus some to serve
- 3 tbsp tikka masala curry paste
- 100g breadcrumbs
- 50g crispy onions
- veg oil, for drizzling

1 Cut the chicken thighs into nugget-sized pieces then put in a bowl with the yogurt and curry paste. Cover and leave in the fridge to marinate for 2 hrs.

2 Heat the oven to 200C/180C fan/gas 6. In a baking dish mix together the breadcrumbs and dried onions. Turn the marinated chicken pieces in the breadcrumb mix then put on a baking tray and drizzle each nugget with some oil (this will help them to get crispy). Roast for 25 mins.

OPTIONAL
Serve the nuggets with mayonnaise swirled with lime zest and mango chutney and some lime wedges.

Nutrition per serving
Kcals 523 • fat 28g • saturates 3g • carbs 34g • sugars 12g • fibre 1g • protein 33g • salt 1.4g

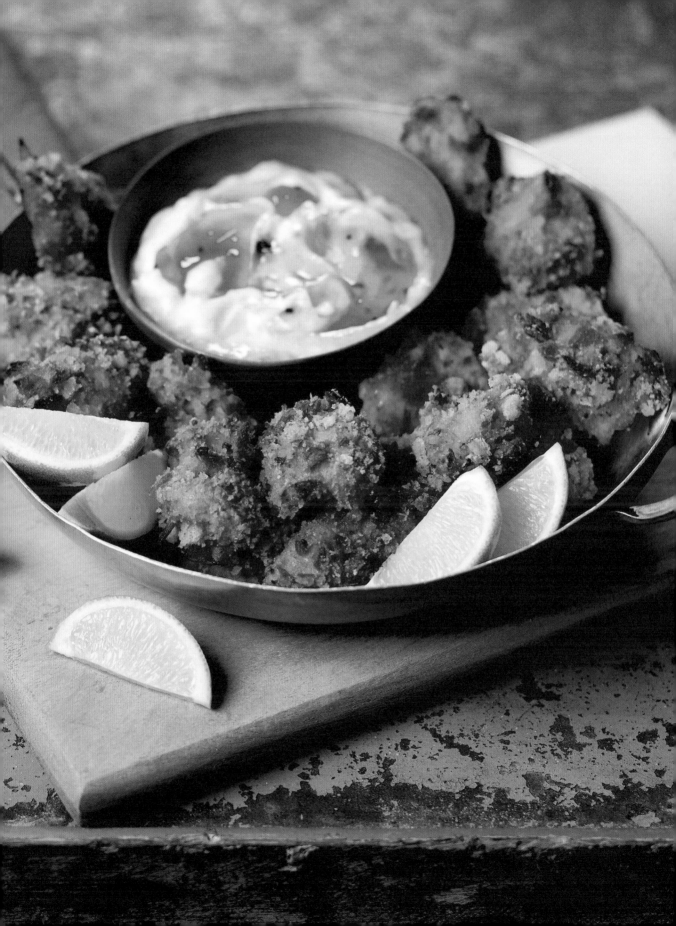

Chicken legs with pesto, kale & butter beans

Prep this chicken dish with pesto, kale and butter beans in 5 minutes and with just 5 main ingredients. It makes a great family weeknight dish.

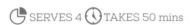 SERVES 4 TAKES 50 mins

- 1 tbsp olive oil
- 4 skin-on chicken legs
- 2 x 400g cans butter beans, drained
- 4 tbsp good-quality pesto
- 100ml white wine
- 180g kale, woody stalks removed

1 Heat a splash of oil in a large frying pan over a medium-high heat, season the chicken and add to the pan skin-side down. Brown for 7–10 mins until the skin is golden and crisp. Meanwhile, mix the butter beans with the pesto, wine and 100ml water. Flip the chicken legs over so that the crispy side is facing up and pour the butter bean mix around them (be careful not to pour over the chicken so that the skin remains crisp).

2 Turn the heat down to a simmer and cook for 20–30 mins until the liquid has reduced by about half and the chicken is cooked through. Remove the meat, set aside and cover with foil. Add the kale to the butter beans, season and cook for 3–5 mins until wilted. Add a splash more water if it looks too dry. Split among 4 plates, top with the crispy chicken legs and crack over some black pepper. Add an extra spoonful of pesto, if you like.

Nutrition per serving
Kcals 626 • fat 34g • saturates 8g • carbs 17g • sugars 3g • fibre 11g • protein 53g • salt 0.7g

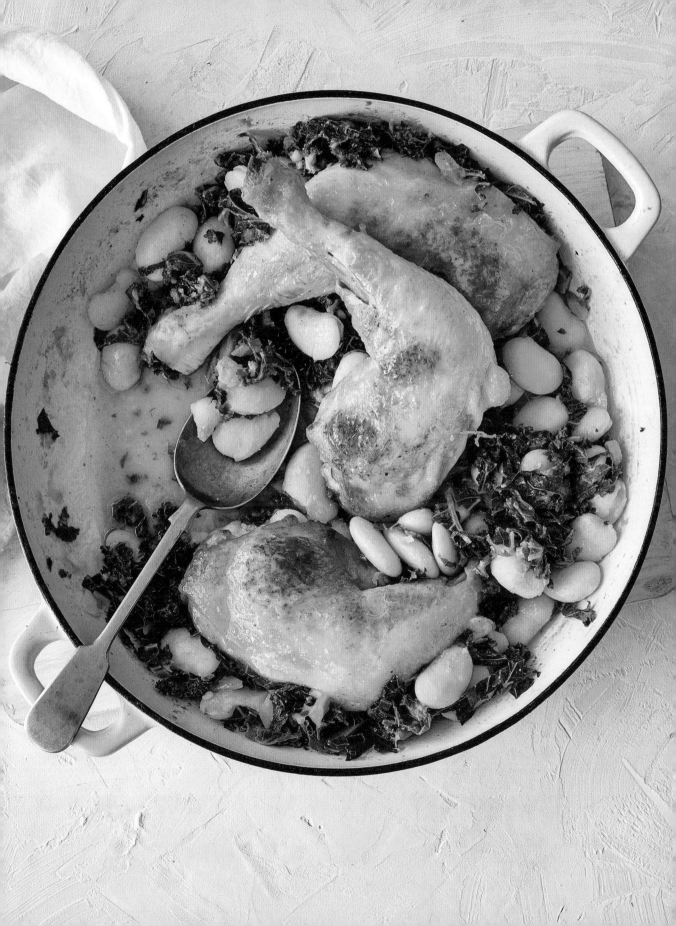

Nutty chicken grain salad

If you're looking for a salad to fill you up, give this easy chicken salad a go. Made with just a handful of ingredients it's perfect when you're short on time.

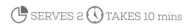 SERVES 2 ⏱ TAKES 10 mins

- 2 chicken breasts
- 2½ tbsp olive oil
- 250g pouch mixed grains
- 100g mixed fruit and nuts
- 100g hummus

1 Put the chicken breasts on a baking tray, drizzle with 1 tbsp olive oil, add seasoning and place under a hot grill for 10 mins, turning after 5, or until cooked through. Meanwhile, heat the grains following pack instructions.
2 Roughly chop the fruit and nuts. Mix with the grains, 1 tbsp olive oil and seasoning to taste. Mix the hummus with 1 tbsp water, ½ tbsp olive oil and some seasoning. Serve the chicken sliced with the grains and drizzle over the hummus dressing.

Nutrition per serving
Kcals 891 • fat 50g • saturates 5g • carbs 55g • sugars 19g • fibre 9g • protein 49g • salt 0.7g

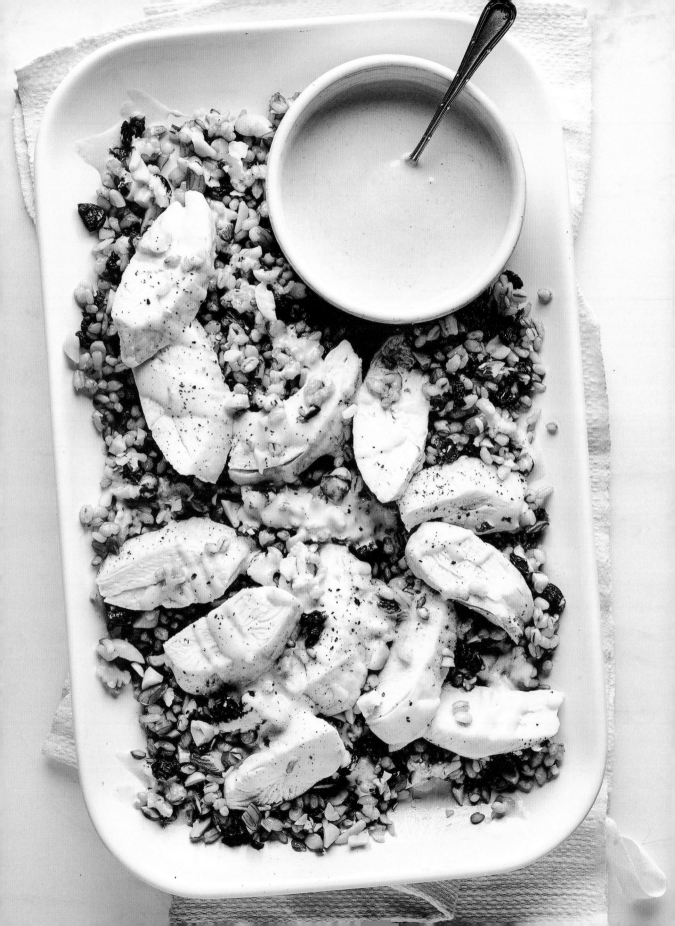

Garlic chicken parcels

Rustle up our chicken parcels with ready-made puff pastry and garlic cream cheese. It's a speedy yet special midweek dinner that only needs a handful ingredients.

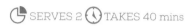 SERVES 2 TAKES 40 mins

- 2 chicken breasts
- 320g sheet all-butter puff pastry
- 150g Boursin or garlic and herb cream cheese
- ½ lemon, zested and cut into wedges, to serve
- 1 tbsp olive oil, plus extra for brushing
- green beans or broccoli, to serve

1 Heat oven to 220C/200C fan/gas 7. Cut a slit halfway in each chicken breast, then put each between 2 pieces of baking parchment and bash out with a rolling pin to flatten slightly.
2 Cut your sheet of pastry in half widthways and put both halves on a baking tray. Sit a chicken breast on top of each half, then cram the cavities with the Boursin (don't worry if a bit of cheese oozes out).
3 Season, scatter over the lemon zest then fold the edges of the pastry in to the centre and pinch shut. Flip each parcel over so the seal is on the bottom. Brush with a little oil, then bake for 30 mins until deep golden.
4 About 10 mins before your parcels are ready, steam or boil the greens until tender. Toss in the oil and season. Serve alongside your chicken parcels with lemon wedges for squeezing over.

Nutrition per serving
Kcals 1115 • fat 80g • saturates 41g • carbs 57g • sugars 6g • fibre 8g • protein 48g • salt 2.4g

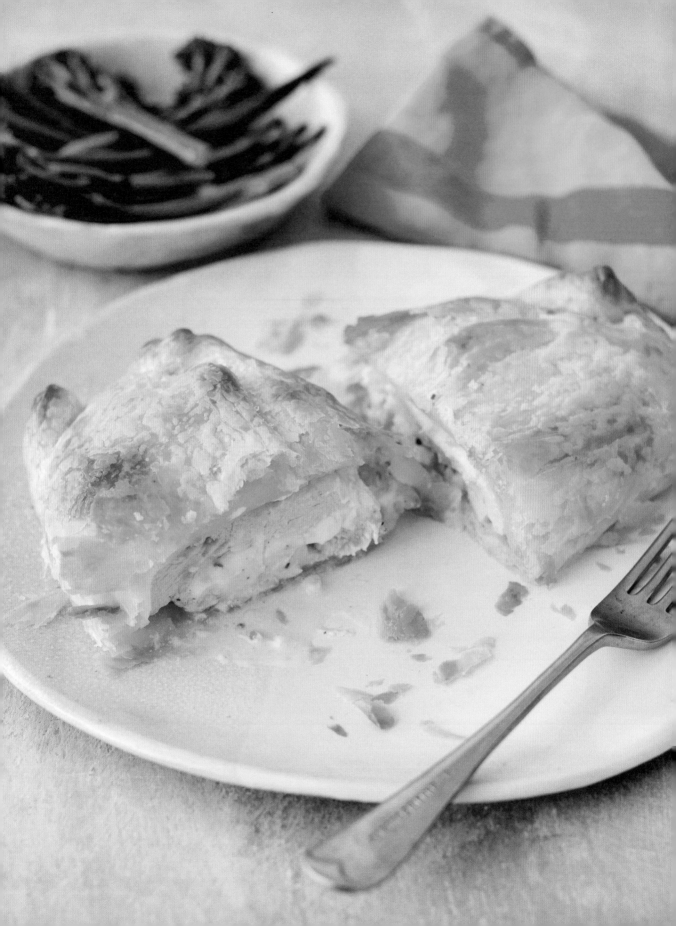

Slow cooker roast chicken

Cooking a chicken in a slow cooker makes it very succulent and packed full of flavour. This simple, freezable recipe is perfect for feeding a family.

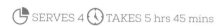 SERVES 4 TAKES 5 hrs 45 mins

- 1 large onion, peeled and cut into thick slices
- 2 carrots, halved lengthways and chopped
- 1 small or medium chicken
- 2 tbsp butter, softened
- 1 bay leaf

1 Heat the slow cooker if necessary. Put the onion and carrot in the base of the stock pot to form a protective layer to sit the chicken on, and add 100ml boiling water. Gently ease the chicken skin away from the breast. Stir some salt and pepper into the butter and push the butter under the skin. Put the bay leaf in the cavity of the chicken and sit on top of the onion and carrot.

2 Cook on low for 5 hrs, then check that the chicken is cooked by wiggling the wing – it should feel very loose. Tip the chicken up so any liquid inside flows out, then cook on high for 30 mins. If the chicken isn't cooked through after the initial time, cook for another hour, then turn the heat up. If you want the skin to be browned, grill it for a couple of minutes (make sure your slow cooker insert is flameproof if you keep it in the pot, or transfer it to a roasting tin).

3 There will be some gravy in the base of the dish with the veg, tip everything through a sieve and press the veg gently to make sure you get every last drop. Serve the veg on the side, if you like.

Nutrition per serving
Kcals 497 • fat 30g • saturates 10g • carbs 7g • sugars 6g • fibre 2g • protein 49g • salt 0.5g

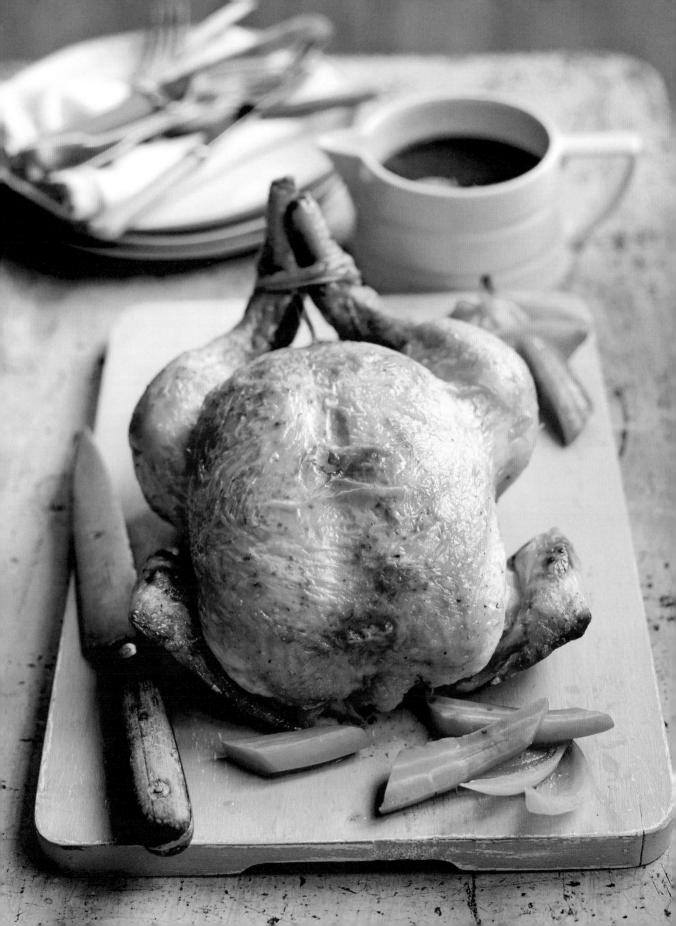

Turkey twist pie

You're just 4 ingredients away from a crispy filo pastry pie, filled with chargrilled veggies, turkey and creamy ricotta. A great low-calorie midweek meal.

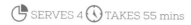 SERVES 4 TAKES 55 mins

- 500g frozen chopped chargrilled vegetables
- 1 tbsp olive oil, plus extra for brushing
- 130g pack roast turkey slices
- 250g tub ricotta
- 270g pack filo pastry (7 sheets)

1 Heat oven to 200C/180C fan/gas 6. Fry the veg in 1 tbsp olive oil for 8–10 mins. Chop the turkey, mix with the veg and ricotta, and season well. Oil a work surface and overlap 4 filo sheets to create a 40 x 60cm rectangle. Brush with oil and layer the remaining sheets on top. Spoon the filling along the bottom third, fold in the short edges, roll up and twist into a spiral. Brush with a little more oil and bake on a non-stick tray for 45 mins.

Nutrition per serving
Kcals 408 • fat 14g • saturates 5g • carbs 47g • sugars 7g • fibre 2g • protein 23g • salt 1.2g

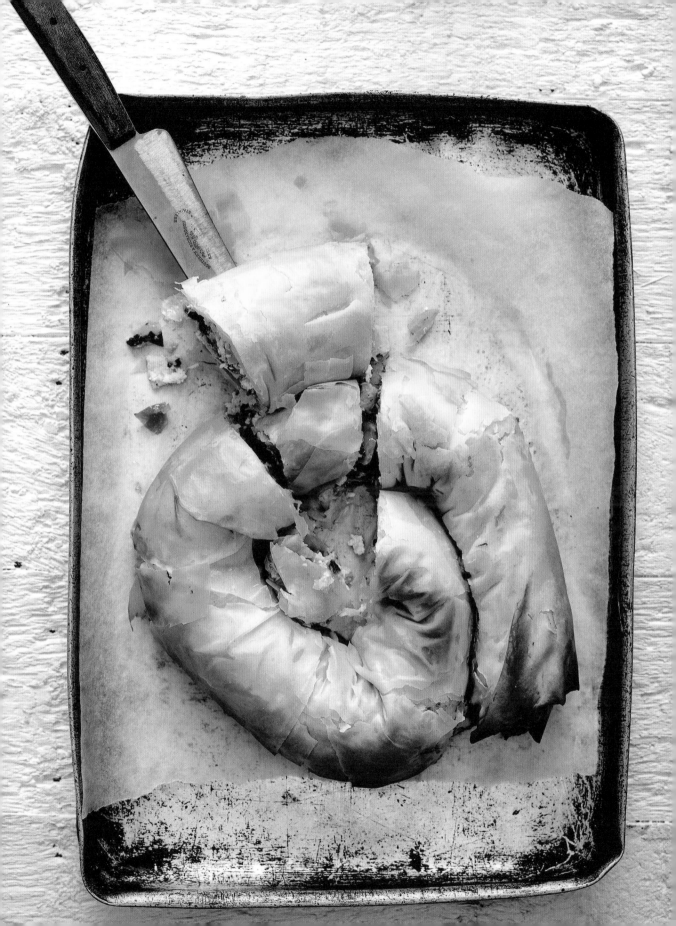

Smoked duck & grilled peach salad

A fruity salad with griddled, caramelised peaches and smoked duck for a light summer lunch.

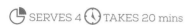 SERVES 4 ⏱ TAKES 20 mins

- 3 tbsp extra virgin olive oil
- 1 tbsp sherry vinegar
- 4 peaches
- 100g watercress
- 50g smoked duck, sliced

1 In a large bowl, mix together the extra virgin olive oil and sherry vinegar with some seasoning.
2 Cut the peaches into quarters and griddle for 2–3 mins each side until charred and slightly caramelised. Toss the watercress with the dressing, then divide among bowls. Top with the peaches and smoked duck.

Nutrition per serving
Kcals 141 • fat 9g • saturates 2g • carbs 8g • sugars 8g • fibre 3g • protein 5g • salt 0.5g

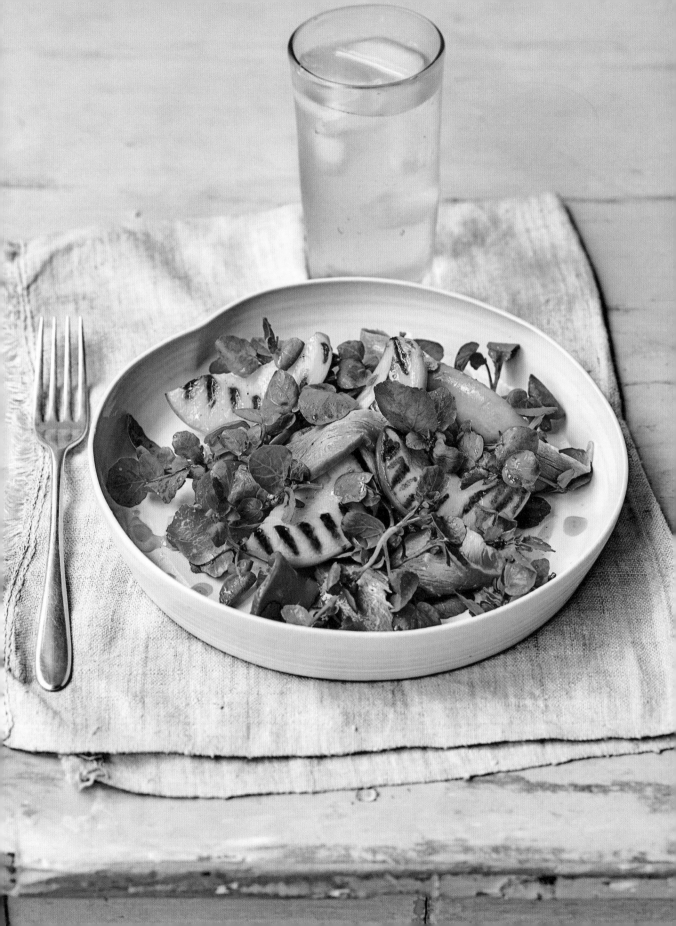

Asparagus & meatball orzo

This springtime pasta dish will be a hit with the whole family. The perfect, fuss-free feast with a creamy sauce and pork meatballs.

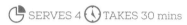 SERVES 4 TAKES 30 mins

- pack 12 pork meatballs
- 500g pack orzo pasta
- large bunch asparagus, woody ends removed, tops sliced in half lengthways
- 200g tub crème fraîche

1 Heat oven to 180C/160C fan/gas 4. Put the meatballs on a tray lined with foil, season and bake for 20 mins until cooked through. Meanwhile, bring a pan of salted water to the boil, add the orzo and cook for 4 mins, then add the asparagus and simmer for 4 mins more. Drain, then tip back into the pan along with the meatballs and crème fraîche, mix and season well.

Nutrition per serving
Kcals 634 • fat 35g • saturates 19g • carbs 37g • sugars 3g • fibre 6g • protein 40g • salt 1.1g

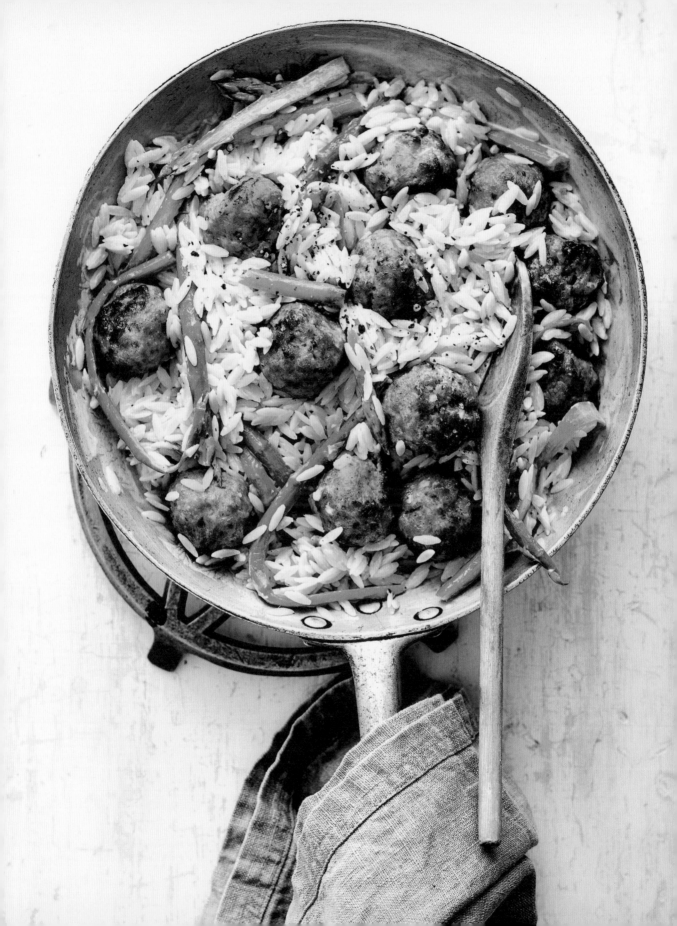

Gammon with watercress & mustard lentils

Rustle up this gluten-free meal of gammon with nutritious watercress and lentils using just 4 ingredients. It's quick and easy but nicely filling.

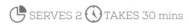 SERVES 2 🕐 TAKES 30 mins

- 1 tbsp olive oil, plus extra for drizzling
- 1 x 250g pouch Puy lentils
- 4 tsp honey mustard dressing
- 100g watercress
- 2 smoked gammon steaks

1 Heat 1 tbsp olive oil in a medium-sized saucepan. Add the lentils, 1 tbsp dressing, ½ the watercress and 150ml water, and cook for 7–8 mins or until the watercress has wilted and the lentils have broken down a little. Season.

2 Heat a griddle pan over a medium heat, drizzle the steaks with oil and cook on each side for 5 mins. Serve with the lentils and the remaining watercress tossed in the rest of the dressing.

Nutrition per serving
Kcals 604 • fat 29g • saturates 7g • carbs 27g • sugars 2g • fibre 10g • protein 55g • salt 6.4g

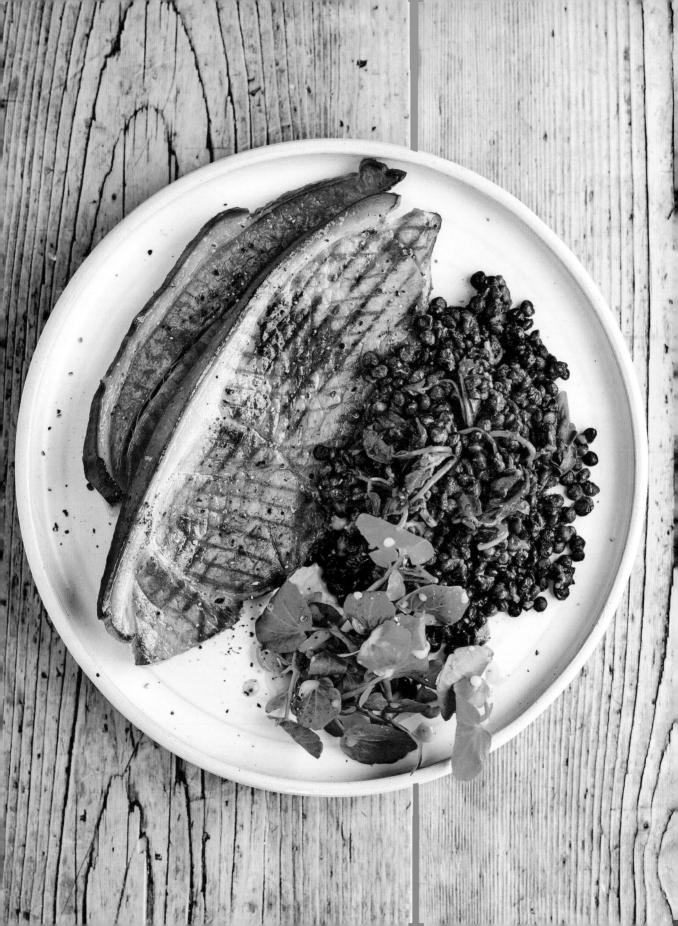

Herby sausages with butter bean mash

A comforting, hearty meal for two with herby sausages and butter bean mash. Just a few ingredients make up this midweek meal that takes just 10 minutes prep.

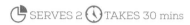 SERVES 2 ⏱ TAKES 30 mins

- 3 tbsp olive oil
- 4 pork and herb sausages
- 8 spring onions, finely sliced
- 2 x 400g cans butter beans, drained and rinsed
- 1 fat garlic clove, finely grated
- zest and juice 1 large lemon

1 Heat grill to high. Brush 1 tbsp oil over the sausages and grill on a tray for 20 mins, turning regularly.

2 Meanwhile, heat the rest of the oil in a saucepan over a low heat. Add most of the spring onion and cook for 5 mins until softened. Add the beans, garlic, and lemon zest and juice, cook for a few mins more, then gently mash with a potato masher to get a thick, creamy consistency. Season and cook for 5 mins more until warmed through. Scatter over the remaining spring onion and serve with the sausages and some wilted greens.

Nutrition per serving
Kcals 617 • fat 36g • saturates 9g • carbs 39g • sugars 5g • fibre 17g • protein 27g • salt 1.2g

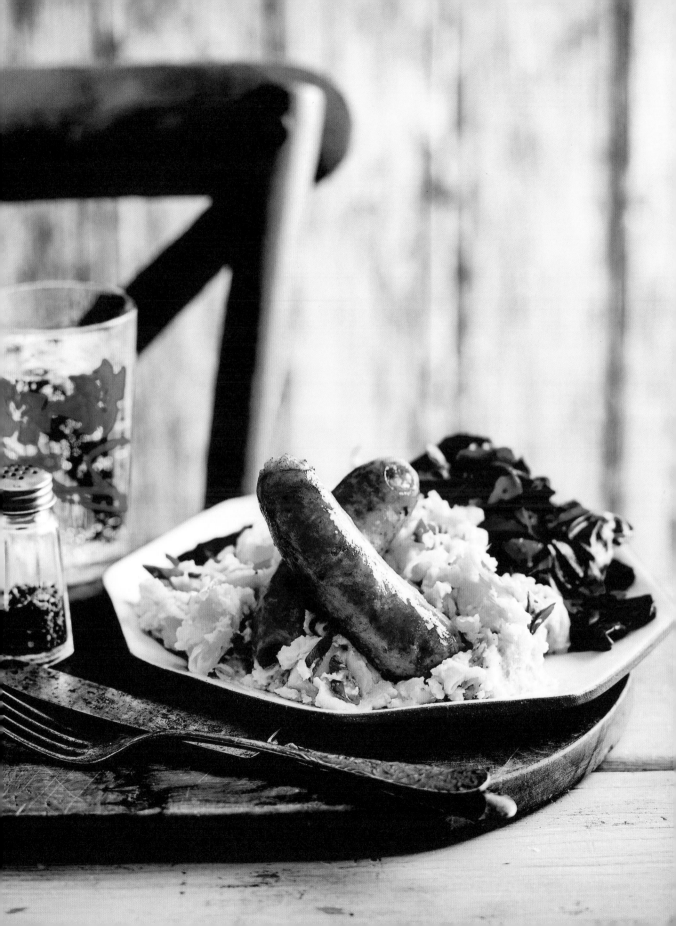

Ultimate chorizo ciabatta

Crusty ciabatta, spicy chorizo, a generous dollop of pesto and sweet roasted peppers make a moreish combination. Serve warm for a quick supper you'll really enjoy.

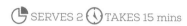 SERVES 2 TAKES 15 mins

- 2 small or 1 large ciabatta
- 150g cooking chorizo, halved lengthways
- 75g pesto
- 200g roasted red peppers from a jar
- handful rocket

1 Heat oven to 180C/160C fan/gas 4 and put the ciabatta in to warm up. Put a griddle pan over a medium heat and cook the chorizo for 5 mins each side or until charred and cooked through.

2 Open up the warmed ciabatta and spread the pesto on the bottom. Layer with the red peppers, then the warm chorizo. Scatter over the rocket, sandwich the ciabatta together, cut in 2 and serve.

Nutrition per serving
Kcals 867 • fat 46g • saturates 12g • carbs 74g • sugars 6g • fibre 6g • protein 37g • salt 4.6g

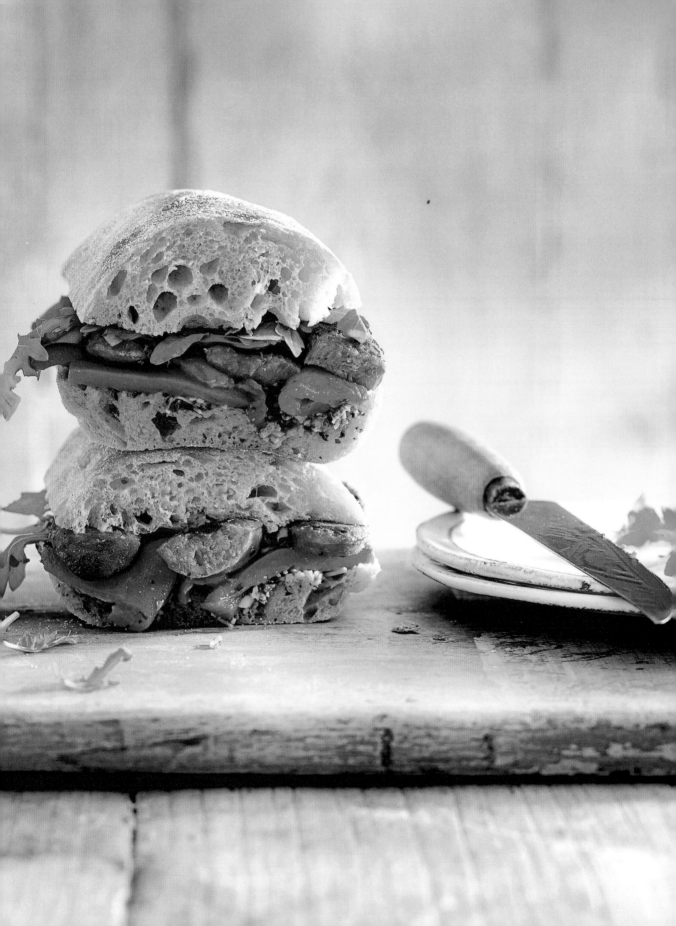

Teriyaki pork meatballs

Pick up these ingredients on your way home for a quick, low-calorie supper. Meatballs in a teriyaki sauce with fresh and crunchy pak choi.

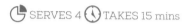 SERVES 4 ⏱ TAKES 15 mins

- 250g dried medium egg noodles
- 2 tbsp sunflower oil
- 12 pork meatballs
- 300g pak choi
- 6 tbsp teriyaki sauce
- ½ lime, juiced

1 Cook the noodles following pack instructions. Add the sunflower oil to a frying pan over a medium heat. Fry the meatballs for 3 mins or until golden brown all over. Lower the heat and cook for 6 mins more. Quarter the pak choi, raise the heat, add the pak choi and cook for 3 mins. Stir through the teriyaki sauce and lime juice, toss everything together with the drained noodles. Divide among bowls and serve.

Nutrition per serving
Kcals 448 • fat 15g • saturates 4g • carbs 50g • sugars 6g • fibre 5g • protein 26g • salt 3.8g

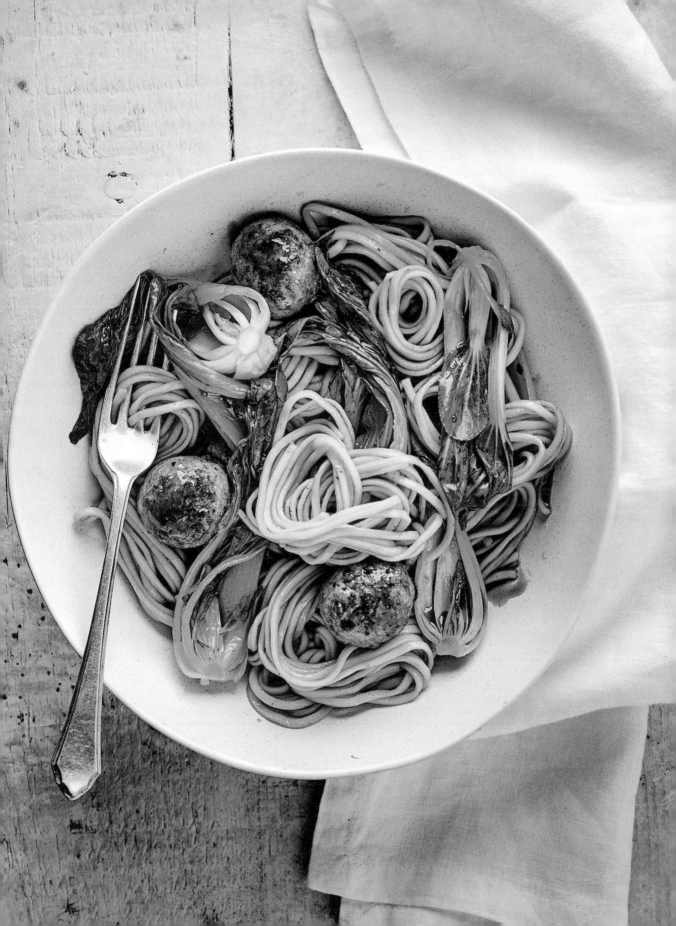

Butter bean & chorizo stew

A hearty stew to feed a family. Spicy chorizo and fresh pesto provide tons of flavour and it's on the table in just 20 minutes.

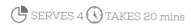 SERVES 4 TAKES 20 mins

- 200g cooking chorizo
- 2 x 400g cans chopped tomatoes
- 2 x 400g cans drained butter beans
- 1 tub fresh pesto
- crusty bread, to serve

1 Slice the chorizo and tip into a large saucepan over a medium heat. Fry gently for 5 mins or until starting to turn dark brown. Add the tomatoes and butter beans, bring to the boil, then simmer for 10 mins. Swirl through the pesto, season lightly and ladle into 4 bowls. Serve with bread for dunking.

Nutrition per serving
Kcals 491 • fat 32g • saturates 8g • carbs 24g • sugars 10g • fibre 8g • protein 23g • salt 2.5g

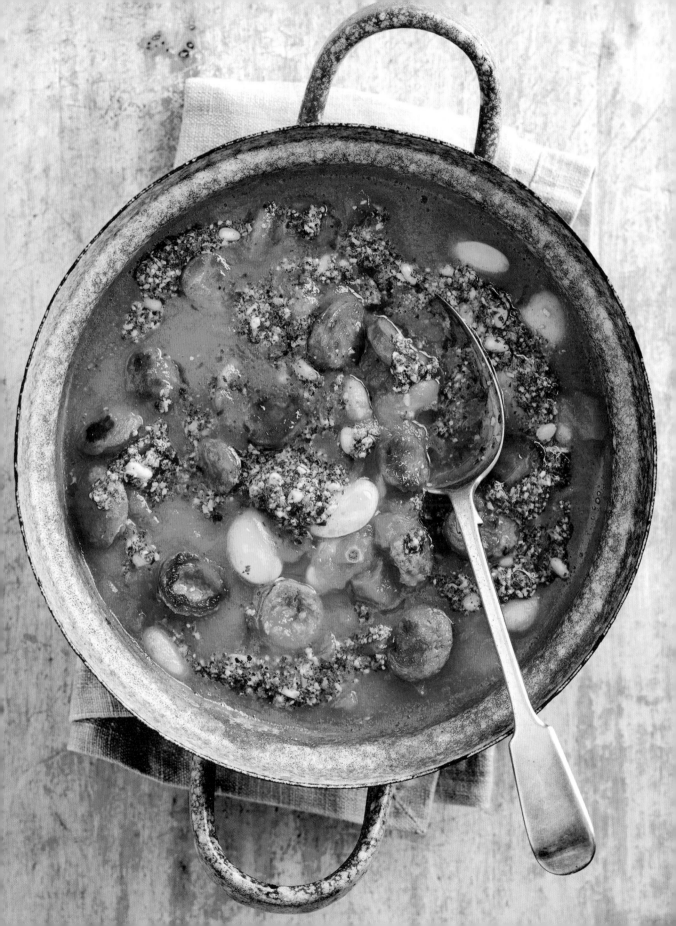

Chorizo & pea risotto

Using simple storecupboard and freezer ingredients, this pea and chorizo risotto makes an easy midweek meal. Garnish with crisped chorizo and grated parmesan.

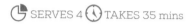 SERVES 4 TAKES 35 mins

- 1 tbsp oil
- 200g chorizo, peeled and chopped
- 300g arborio risotto rice
- 1.2 litres chicken stock (fresh is best), heated until simmering
- 200g frozen peas
- 60g parmesan, finely grated, plus extra to serve

1 Heat the oil in a large frying pan, tip in the chorizo and fry until it is crisp and all the oil has been released. Remove a quarter of the chorizo with a slotted spoon and set aside.

2 Tip the rice into the pan, stir to coat it in the oil and toast for a min or so. Add a ladleful of the stock, stir then, once absorbed, add a bit more. Continue doing this for about 20 mins until most of the stock has been absorbed and the rice has swollen but still has a slight bite.

3 Tip in the peas, parmesan and the remaining stock. Give everything a good stir. Once the cheese has melted, season with black pepper, then divide among bowls, topping each portion with the remaining crisp chorizo and extra grated parmesan.

Nutrition per serving
Kcals 642 • fat 25g • saturates 10g • carbs 68g • sugars 4g • fibre 6g • protein 34g • salt 2.8g

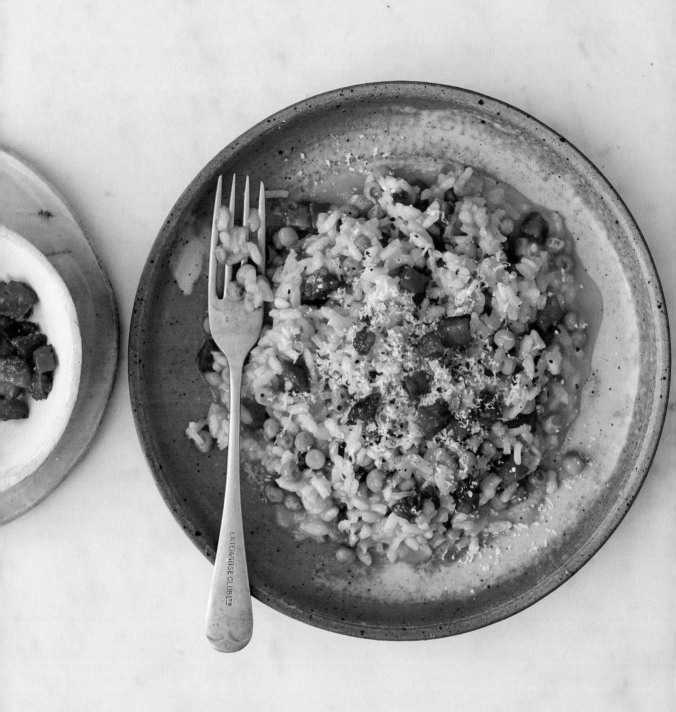

Sausages with pesto mash

Add a generous dollop of pesto to the standard sausage and mash – an easy way to liven up your midweek meal.

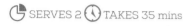 SERVES 2 · TAKES 35 mins

- 3 large white potatoes
- olive oil, for frying
- 4 pork sausages
- 200g cherry tomatoes on the vine
- ½ tub fresh pesto

1 Peel and quarter the potatoes, then cook in a large pan of salted, boiling water for 15 mins. Drain and set aside.
2 Pour a glug of olive oil into a large frying pan over a medium heat and cook the sausages for 15 mins. Add the tomatoes to the pan for the final 5 mins. Mash the potatoes well and mix in the pesto. Season and serve with the sausages and tomatoes.

Nutrition per serving
Kcals 697 · fat 40g · saturates 8g · carbs 65g · sugars 8g · fibre 8g · protein 15g · salt 2.6g

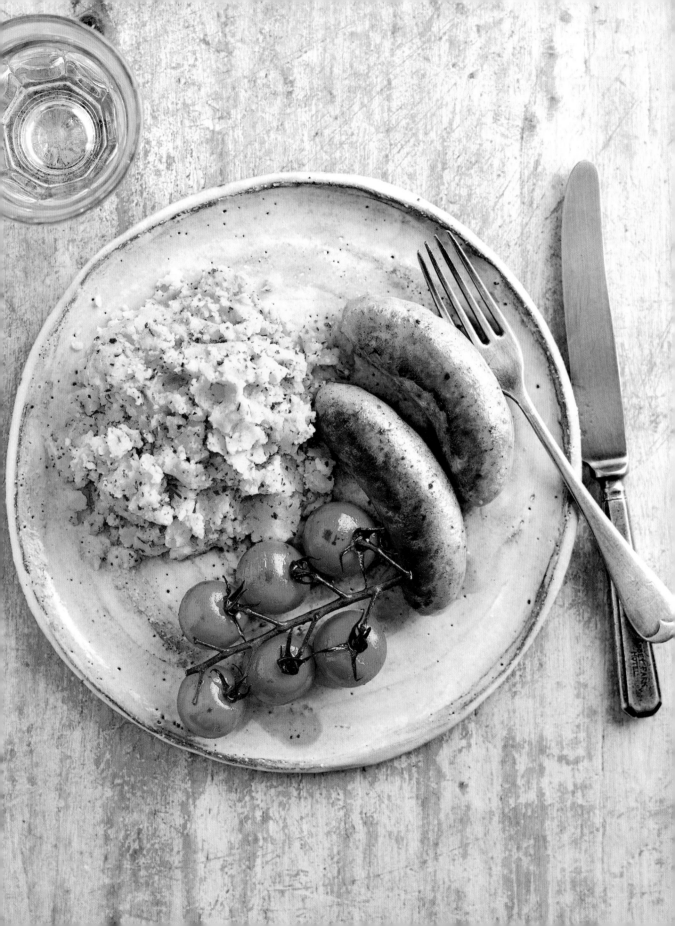

Barbecued lamb with mint chutney

This beautiful barbecued lamb with a fresh minty chutney makes a great sharing dish for friends. Serve with new potatoes and salad.

SERVES 6 · TAKES 1 hr 20 mins plus marinating

- 1 large pack mint (about 100g), leaves picked
- 1 small pack coriander
- 3 garlic cloves
- 1 lemon, juiced
- 1 small leg of lamb, about 1½kg, butterflied (ask your butcher to do this for you)

1 First, make the chutney. Put the mint, coriander, garlic, lemon, a good pinch of salt and a small splash of water in a minichopper or food processor and blitz to a chunky paste. Will keep in the fridge for 2 days.

2 Use a third of the chutney to marinate the lamb for at least a couple of hours, or up to 24 hrs before.

3 To cook the lamb, heat the barbecue until the coals are ashen. Grill the lamb, flesh-side down, for about 25 mins, then flip it over and cook on the fat side for about 15 mins until charred and sizzling. When the lamb is cooked to your liking, leave it to rest on a warm platter to catch the juices. To serve, carve the lamb into thick slices, again catching the juices. In a bowl, mix the cooking juices with the remaining chutney, and serve alongside the lamb.

Nutrition per serving
Kcals 357 · fat 20g · saturates 8g · carbs 1g · sugars 0.1g · fibre 0.3g · protein 43g · salt 0.4g

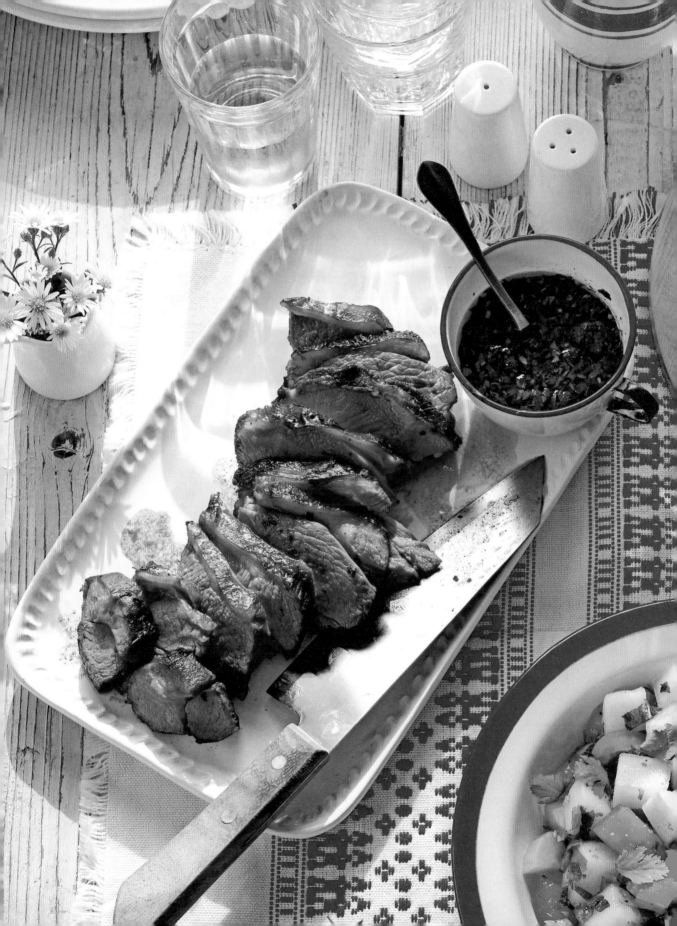

Next level carbonara

Make the ultimate spaghetti carbonara with a creamy hollandaise-style sauce and crisp pancetta or guanciale. You can also mix in an egg yolk at the end.

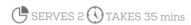 SERVES 2 TAKES 35 mins

- 1 tbsp olive oil
- 150g rindless unsmoked fatty pancetta or guanciale, finely chopped
- 1 garlic clove, bashed
- 200g spaghetti or fettuccine
- 4 good-quality egg yolks, (2 of them are optional)
- 50g parmesan, finely grated

1 First, warm your serving dishes in a low oven or in the microwave. Heat the oil gently in a large, shallow pan. Fry the guanciale or pancetta and garlic for 10 mins, or until all the fat has rendered off and the meat is golden and crisp. Remove and discard the garlic clove, then turn off the heat.

2 Bring a large pan of salted water to a simmer and cook the pasta until it's al dente (about a minute less than the pack instructions). Meanwhile, whisk 2 egg yolks in a small bowl with a pinch of salt.

3 Using kitchen tongs, lift the pasta from the water into the pancetta pan along with any dripping water. Use a wooden spoon to stir it into the rendered fat. If the pan looks dry, add a small ladleful of pasta water and mix it in. Keep adding until you see a little pasta water at the bottom of the pan – you'll be surprised how much will be absorbed.

4 Working quickly, tip the beaten yolks in with the pasta and stir vigorously. Rinse the yolk bowl out with a little more pasta water and pour that in too. Add most of the parmesan and beat again. If at any time it's becoming claggy or starting to scramble, pour in a little more water. If you've added too much, stir the pasta over the lowest heat for a few moments. You're aiming for a smooth sauce that is the consistency of double cream. Season with a couple of pinches of ground black pepper and taste for salt.

5 Transfer the pasta to the warmed serving dishes, scatter over the remaining parmesan and nestle the last 2 egg yolks on top, if using. Season them with some salt and pepper and serve.

Nutrition per serving
Kcals 757 • fat 42g • saturates 15g • carbs 55g • sugars 2g • fibre 3g • protein 37g • salt 3g

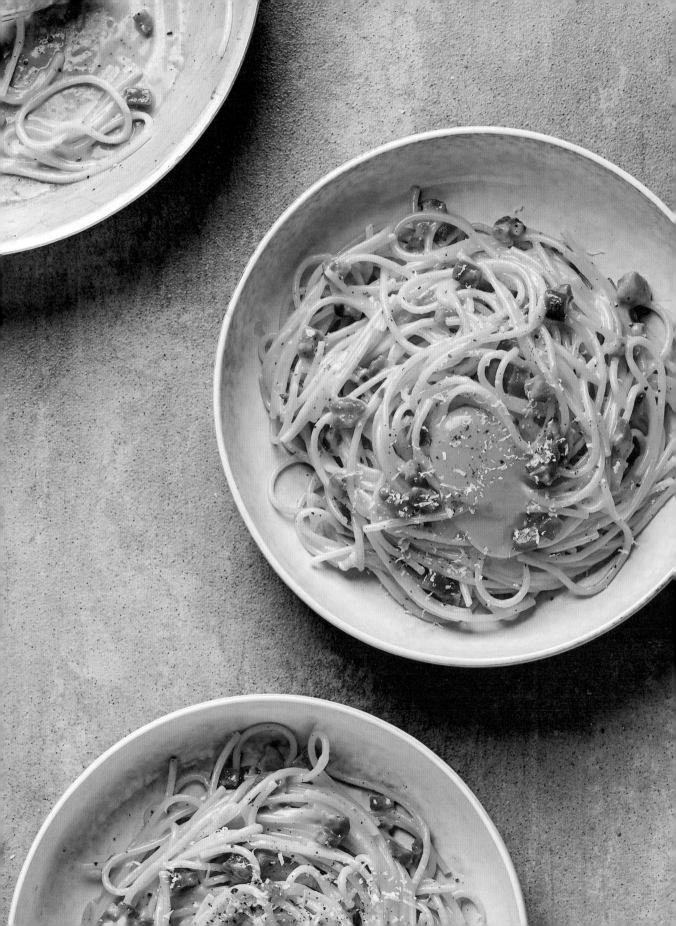

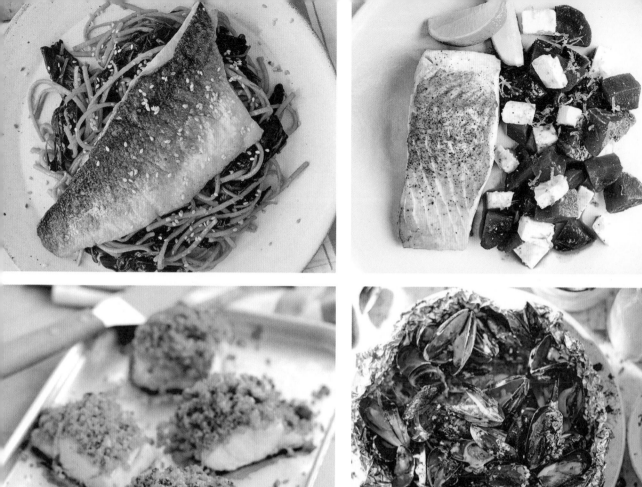

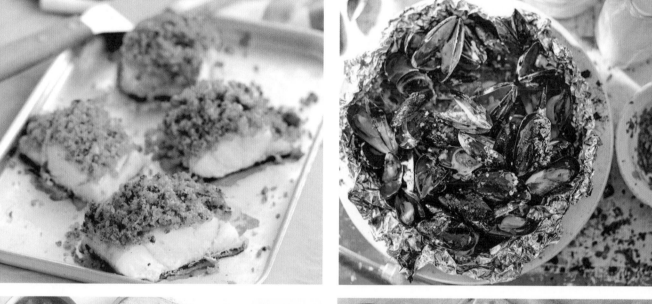

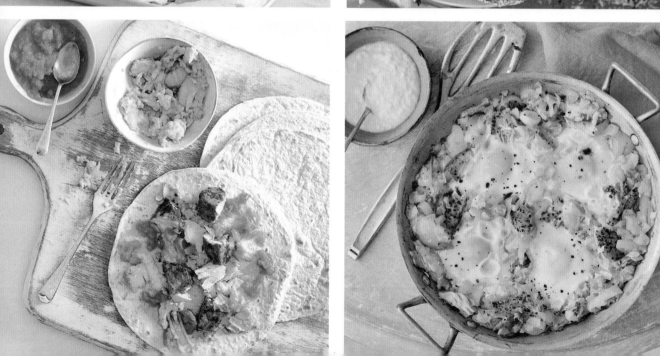

CHAPTER 6: FISH & SEAFOOD

Fish (especially the oily varieties) is so good for us, and most of us should be eating more of it. This chapter will make it much easier to do just that, with healthy, simple recipes you can make in no time at all. Neighbourhood fishmongers are wonderful if you have one, but supermarket fish counters are becoming just as well stocked and knowledgeable. It's often cheaper to buy a whole large fish, such as salmon, and ask the fishmonger to fillet it for you than buying individual fillets. You can store them in the freezer for a few months ready for whenever you want to whip up one of these simple dinners.

Blackened salmon fajitas

In need of a quick fix? Go Tex-Mex with these fish fajitas that'll feed 4 in 15 minutes!

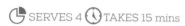 SERVES 4 ⏱ TAKES 15 mins

- 4 salmon fillets
- sunflower oil, or any oil suitable for frying
- 1 fajita kit
- 2 avocados
- 2 limes

1 Coat the salmon in 1 tbsp oil and the fajita spice mix. Add 1 tbsp oil to a frying pan and fry for 8 mins until blackened.
2 Mash the avocados with a fork, season and squeeze over the juice of 1 lime and some salt. Serve the salmon in large flakes with the tortillas, avocado, salsa and the other lime, cut into wedges.

Nutrition per serving
Kcals 759 • fat 45g • saturates 10g • carbs 46g • sugars 8g • fibre 7g • protein 39g • salt 2g

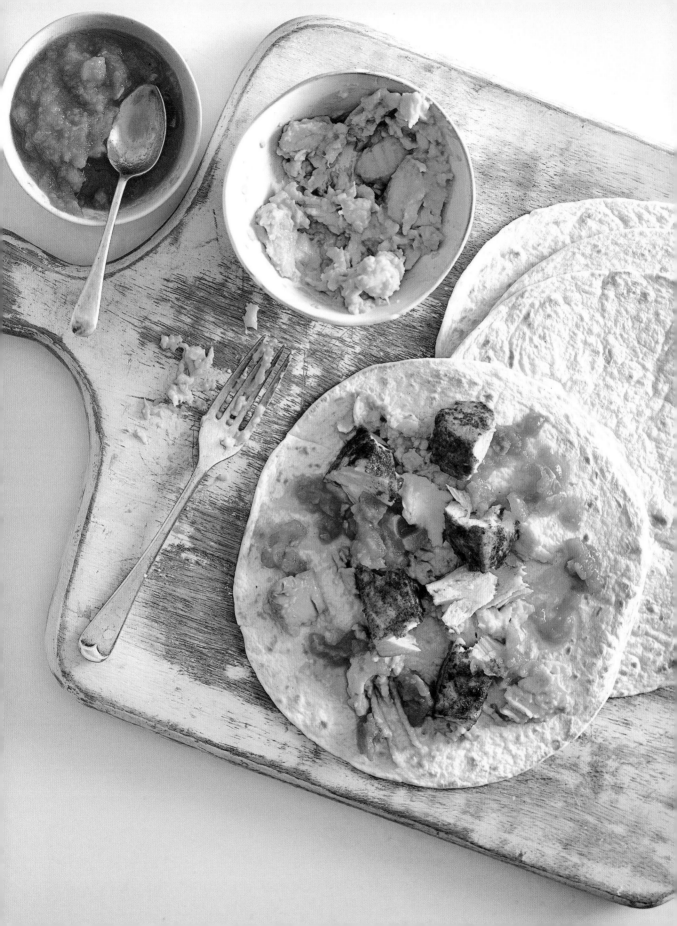

Jerk prawn & coconut rice bowl

Within just a matter of minutes you can cook up a filling coconut rice bowl with king prawns – simple, speedy, nice and spicy!

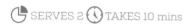 SERVES 2 TAKES 10 mins

- 1 tbsp flavourless oil
- 150g pack raw peeled king prawns
- 1½ tbsp jerk seasoning
- 400g can kidney beans in chilli sauce
- 250g pouch coconut rice
- ½ lime, cut into wedges

1 Heat the oil in a large frying pan. Add the prawns and the jerk seasoning, and cook for 1–2 mins. Drain the beans, reserving 3 tbsp of the chilli sauce.

2 Add the beans to the pan along with the reserved sauce and the coconut rice. Fry for 3–4 mins, then season with salt to taste and spoon into 2 bowls, squeeze over the lime juice and serve.

Nutrition per serving
Kcals 531 • fat 14g • saturates 5g • carbs 62g • sugars 11g • fibre 13g • protein 29g • salt 2.6g

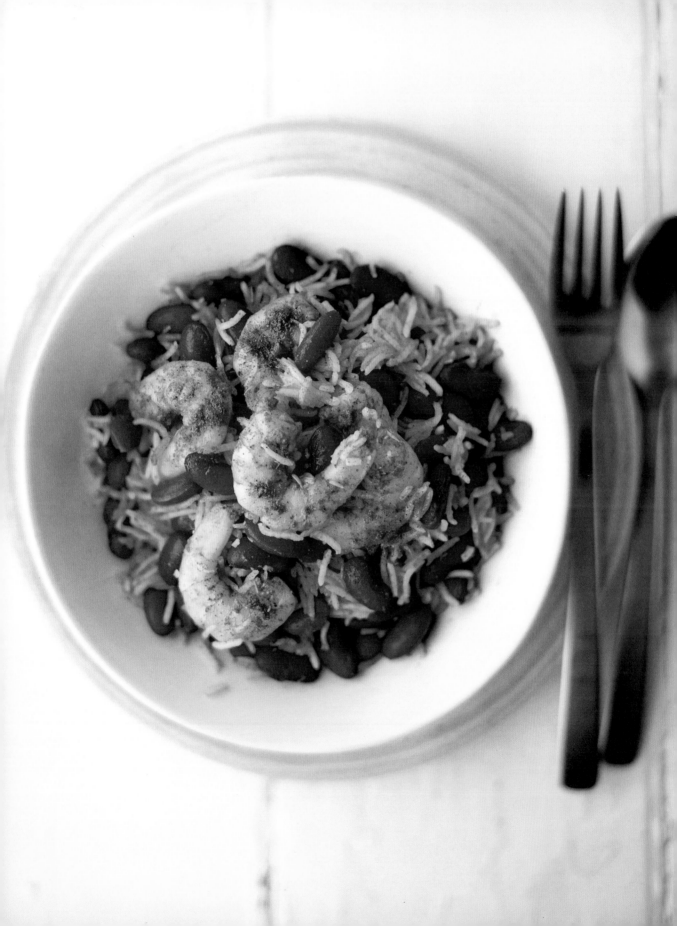

White fish with sesame noodles

Whip up this tasty seabass served with spinach, noodles and sesame seeds in just 20 minutes. It makes a great choice if you're looking for a speedy supper.

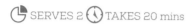 SERVES 2 ◷ TAKES 20 mins

- 25g toasted sesame seeds, plus extra to serve
- 2 tbsp soy sauce
- 1 tbsp sesame oil, plus a drizzle
- 150g soba or wholemeal noodles (300g if using pre-cooked)
- 200g bag spinach
- 2 seabass fillets

1 Use a spice grinder or pestle and mortar to crush the sesame seeds, then stir in the soy sauce, oil and 1 tbsp of water to make a creamy dressing, season and set aside.

2 Bring a pan of salted water to the boil, add the noodles and cook following pack instructions, then drain and set aside. Using the same pan, tip in all the spinach and cook until reduced down and dark green. Tip in the noodles, along with the sesame dressing and a splash of water and toss well to heat through.

3 Heat a drizzle of oil in a non-stick frying pan over a medium to high heat. Season the skin of the seabass, then place in the pan skin-side down, fry until the skin has crisped up and the flesh has nearly all turned opaque, around 3 mins. Flip over and fry for 30 seconds further, until the fish is flaking and cooked through. Divide the noodles and greens between 2 bowls and place the fish on top. Scatter over the toasted sesame seeds and serve.

Nutrition per serving
Kcals 624 • fat 24g • saturates 4g • carbs 54g • sugars 3g • fibre 7g • protein 45g • salt 4.1g

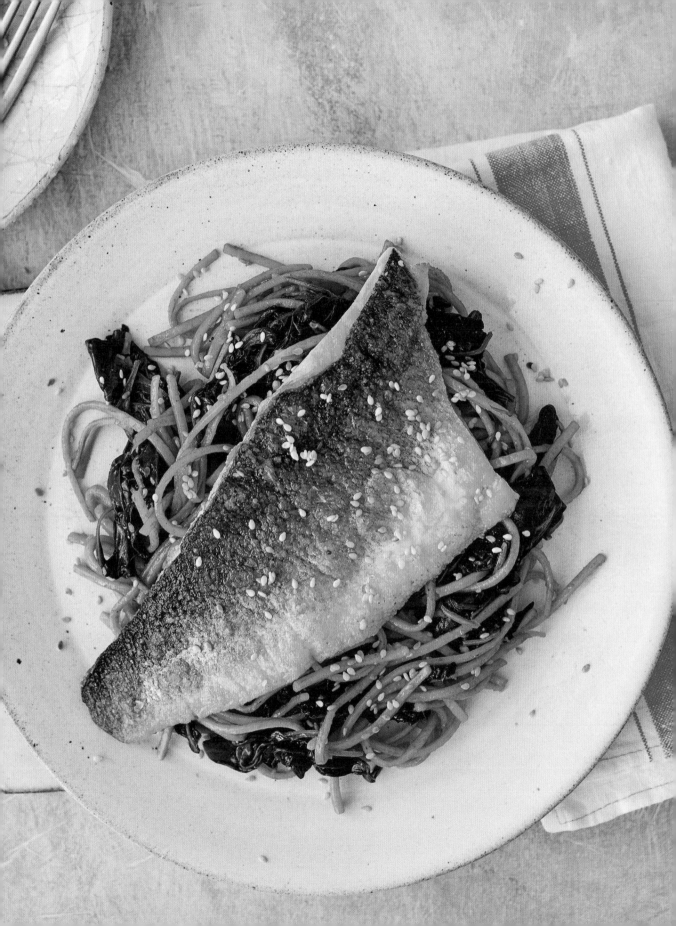

Hoisin mackerel pancakes

Need a speedy, DIY family meal? Try these mackerel pancakes. Using sweet ingredients with stronger-flavoured fish such as mackerel helps tempt children to try them.

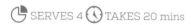 SERVES 4 TAKES 20 mins

- 3 mackerel fillets, all bones removed, cut into finger-length strips
- 2 tbsp hoisin sauce, plus extra for dipping
- 4 spring onions or ½ cucumber, or both
- 2 Little Gem lettuces
- 1 tsp vegetable oil
- 10 Chinese pancakes

1 Marinate the mackerel in the hoisin sauce while you prepare the veg. Cut the spring onions and cucumber into thin matchsticks, and separate the lettuce leaves.

2 Heat the oil in a large frying pan over a medium heat. Add the mackerel and fry for 3–4 mins until sticky and caramelised. Heat the pancakes following pack instructions. Serve everything in the middle of the table and let everyone help themselves.

Nutrition per serving
Kcals 393 • fat 22g • saturates 4g • carbs 24g • sugars 9g • fibre 3g • protein 24g • salt 0.9g

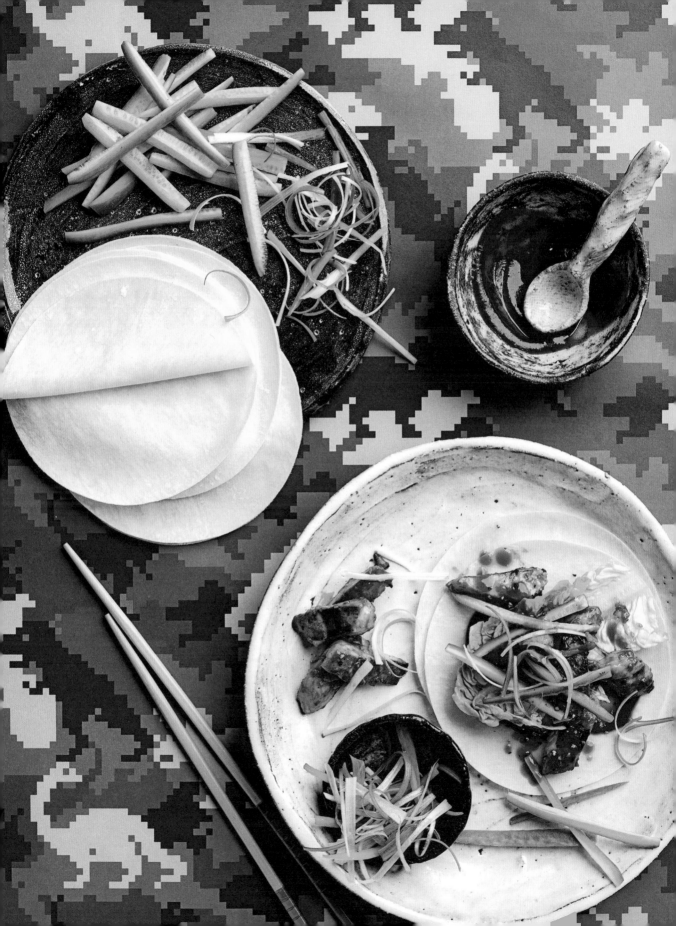

One-pot coconut fish curry

Cook our easy one-pot curry in just half an hour, with only 5 mins prep. It's ideal for feeding the family quickly, on a budget. Serve with rice and yogurt.

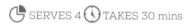 SERVES 4 ⏱ TAKES 30 mins

- 1 tbsp sunflower oil, vegetable oil or coconut oil
- 1 onion, chopped
- 2 tbsp curry paste, we used korma
- 400ml can coconut milk
- 390g pack fish pie mix
- 200g frozen peas

1 Heat the oil in a large saucepan over a medium heat, add the onion and a big pinch of salt. Gently fry until the onion is translucent, so around 10 mins, then add the curry paste. Stir and cook for another minute. Tip in the coconut milk and stir well, then simmer for 10 mins.

2 Tip the fish pie mix and the frozen peas into the pan and cook until the peas are bright green and the fish is starting to flake, so around 3 mins. Ladle into bowls and serve with limes wedges, yogurt and rice.

Nutrition per serving
Kcals 371 • fat 25g • saturates 16g • carbs 12g • sugars 7g • fibre 5g • protein 23g • salt 0.8g

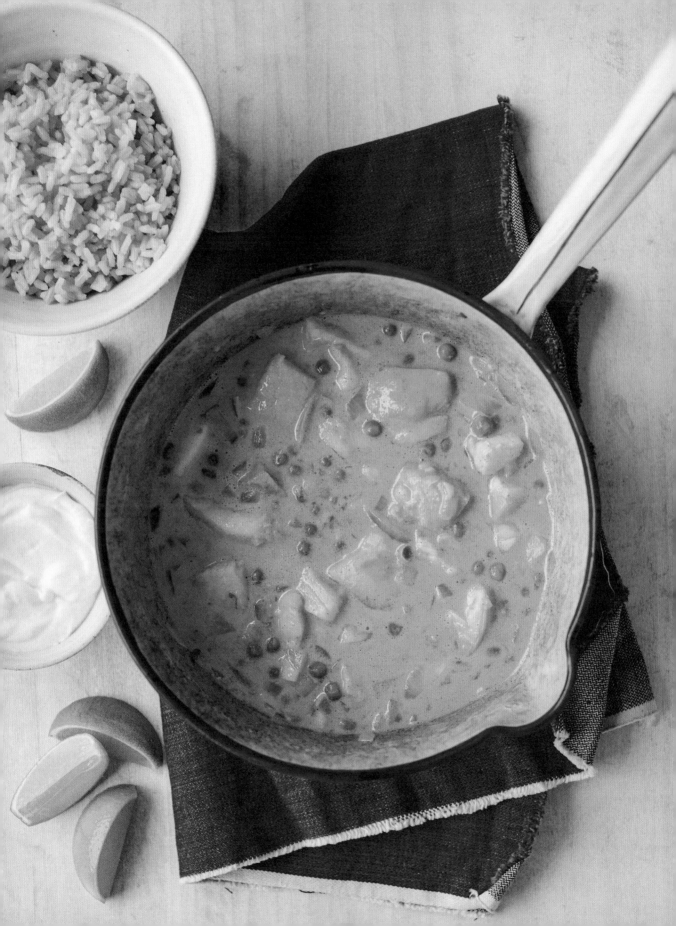

Easy laksa

A super-quick version of this flavoursome Thai soup.

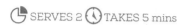 SERVES 2 TAKES 5 mins

- 3 tbsp Thai green curry paste
- 400ml can coconut milk
- 150g cooked prawns
- 250g courgettes, peeled into ribbons or spiralized
- ½ lime, juiced

1 Cook the curry paste for 1 min in a saucepan, adding a splash of water if it sticks. Pour in the coconut milk, then leave to bubble away for a few mins before adding the prawns, courgette and lime. Cook for 1 min more to warm through, then divide between bowls.

Nutrition per serving
Kcals 478 • fat 39g • saturates 29g • carbs 11g • sugars 7g • fibre 4g • protein 18g • salt 2.1g

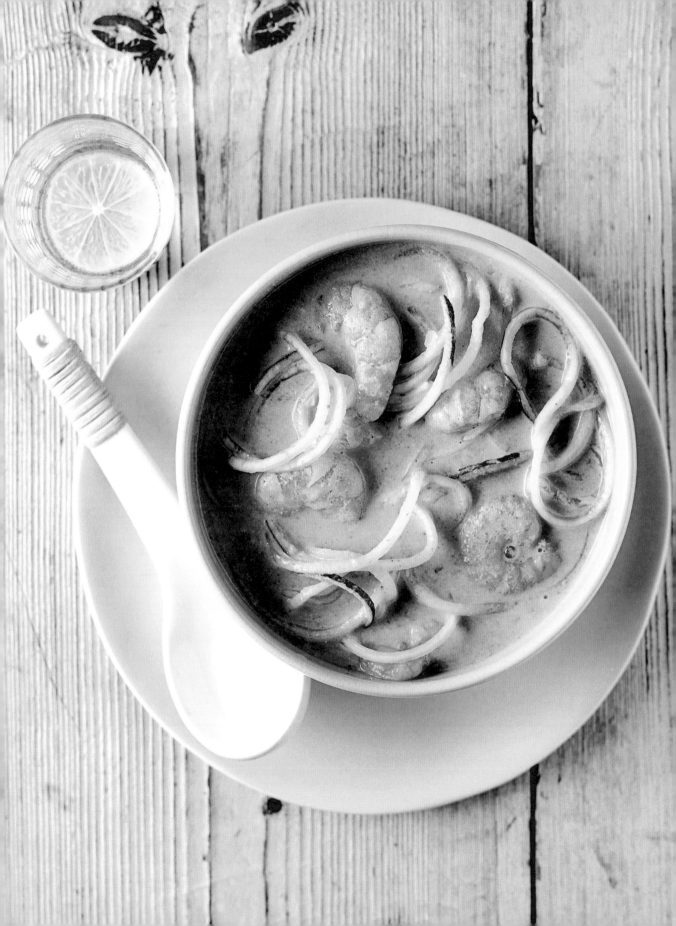

Salmon with beetroot, feta & lime salsa

Rustle up this tasty salmon dish, ideal for a quick and easy midweek meal with a tasty feta and beetroot salsa on the side.

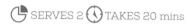 SERVES 2 ⏱ TAKES 20 mins

- 200g cooked beetroot
- 70g feta
- 2 limes
- 2 tbsp olive oil
- 2 skin-on salmon fillets

1 Chop the beetroot and feta into small cubes and mix with the juice and zest of 1 lime, 1 tbsp oil and some seasoning.

2 Season the salmon. Heat the remaining oil in a non-stick frying pan over a high heat. When hot add the salmon, skin-side down, and cook for 3 mins. Flip over, turn the heat down and cook for a further 4–5 mins. Serve with the beetroot salsa and the remaining lime, cut into wedges.

Nutrition per serving
Kcals 556 • fat 39g • saturates 9g • carbs 12g • sugars 10g • fibre 4g • protein 36g • salt 1.2g

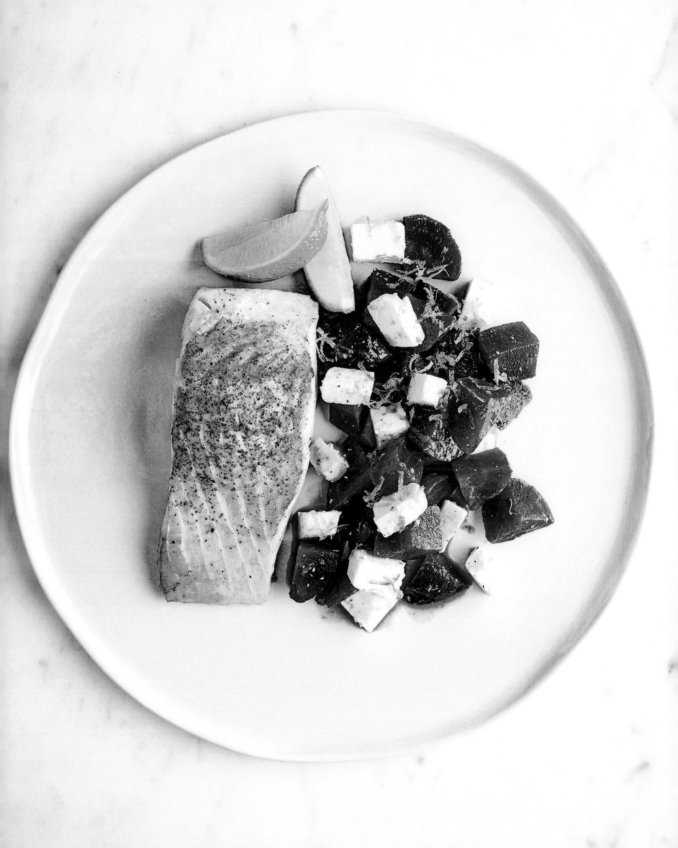

Prawn & leek frittata

Omelettes step aside, this frittata is a speedy weeknight lifesaver that's packed with flavour and goes well with salad or crusty bread.

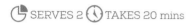 SERVES 2 🕐 TAKES 20 mins

- 2 tbsp olive oil
- 3 large leeks
- 150g pack raw peeled king prawns
- 5 large eggs
- 120g garlic and herb cream cheese
- salad or crusty bread, to serve

1 Heat the olive oil in a medium frying pan. Slice the leeks and add to the pan, cooking for 5 mins. Add the prawns and cook for 1 min more. Beat the eggs and whisk through half the cream cheese. Season to taste. Pour the mixture over the prawns and leeks, dot over the remaining cheese and cook on a medium heat for 5–8 mins. Finish under a medium-hot grill for 2 mins until just set with a slight wobble.

Nutrition per serving
Kcals 476 • fat 30g • saturates 9g • carbs 10g • sugars 8g • fibre 7g • protein 37g • salt 1.6g

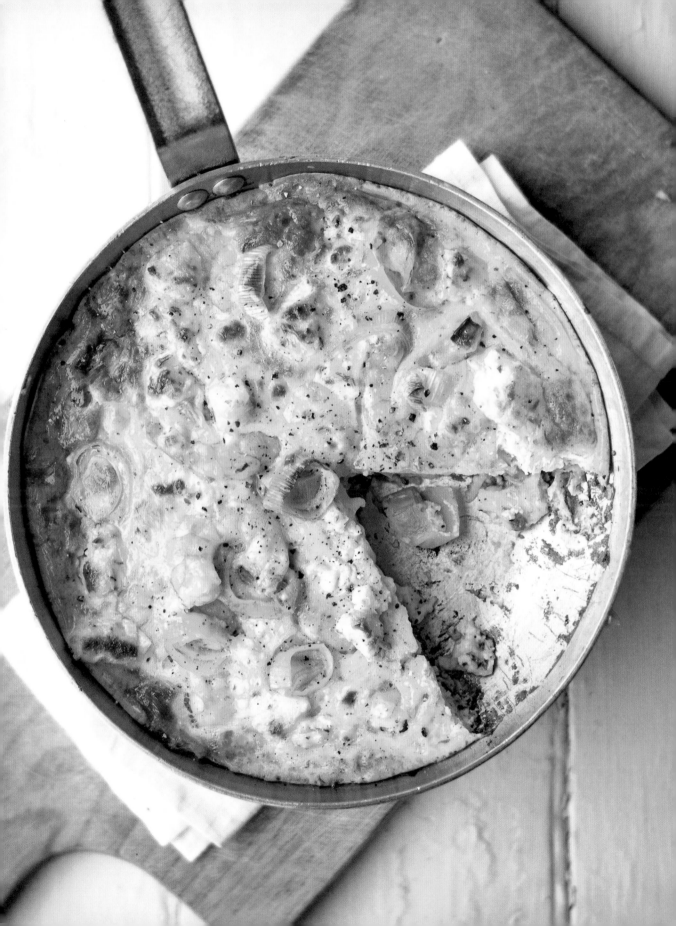

Smoked mackerel & leek hash with horseradish

Make this mackerel and leek hash in just 30 minutes. It uses just a few ingredients and can be served in the pan, so makes a great choice on busy weeknights.

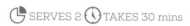 SERVES 2 TAKES 30 mins

- 250g new potatoes, halved
- 2 tbsp oil
- 2 large leeks, thinly sliced
- 4 eggs
- 100g peppered smoked mackerel, skin removed
- 2 tbsp creamed horseradish

1 Put the potatoes in a microwaveable bowl with a splash of water, cover, then cook on high for 5 mins until tender (or steam or simmer them).
2 Meanwhile, heat the oil in a frying pan over a medium heat, add the leeks with a pinch of salt and cook for 10 mins, stirring so they don't stick, until softened. Tip in the potatoes, turn up the heat and fry for a couple of mins to crisp them up a bit. Flake through the mackerel.
3 Make 4 indents in the leek mixture in the pan, crack an egg into each, season, then cover the pan and cook for 6–8 mins until the whites have set and the yolks are runny. Serve the horseradish on the side, with the pan in the middle of the table.

Nutrition per serving
Kcals 546 • fat 35g • saturates 6g • carbs 25g • sugars 7g • fibre 7g • protein 29g • salt 1.7g

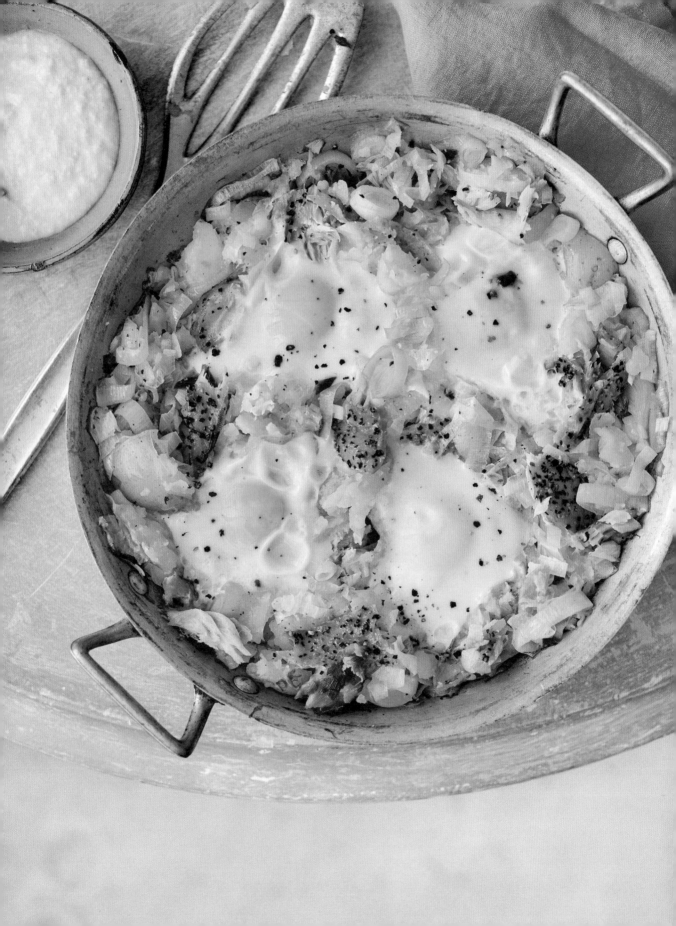

Salmon & spinach pasta

A fresh, healthy pasta dish that's ready in a flash. A handful of punchy ingredients make for a colourful supper that's high in folate, fibre, iron and omega-3.

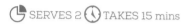 SERVES 2 ⏱ TAKES 15 mins

- 200g penne
- 2 skinless salmon fillets
- 60g sundried tomatoes
- 80g bag spinach
- ½ lemon, juiced

1 Cook the pasta following pack instructions. Fry the salmon for 4–6 mins with the tomatoes in their oil. Flake the fish in the pan, then add the drained pasta, spinach and lemon, season well. Stir for 1–2 mins until the spinach is wilted and everything is coated.

Nutrition per serving
Kcals 811 • fat 24g • saturates 4g • carbs 96g • sugars 14g • fibre 10g • protein 48g • salt 0.4g

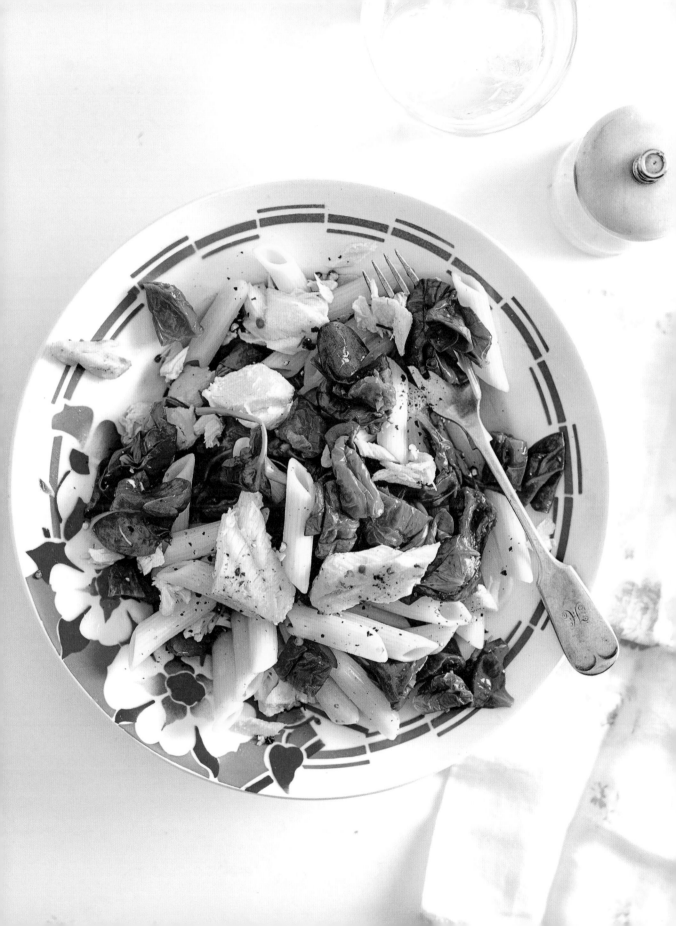

Salmon & ginger fishcakes

Create a complete super-healthy supper with these light, Asian-style fish cakes and sweet potato chips.

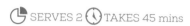 SERVES 2 ⏱ TAKES 45 mins

- 1 large sweet potato, cut into chips
- 4 tsp olive oil
- 2 x 140g skinless salmon fillets
- thumbnail-sized piece ginger, grated
- zest 1 lime, plus wedges to serve
- ½ bunch spring onions, finely chopped

1 Heat oven to 200C/180C fan/gas 6. Toss the chips in a roasting tin with 1 tsp oil. Season and bake for 20–25 mins.
2 Chop the salmon as finely as you can and place in a bowl with the ginger, lime zest and seasoning. Heat 1 tsp oil in a non-stick pan and soften the spring onions for 2 mins. Stir into the salmon, mix well and shape into 4 patties.
3 Heat the remaining oil in the pan and cook the patties for 3–4 mins each side until golden and cooked through. Cover with a lid and leave to rest for a few mins. Serve 2 patties each with the chips and lime wedges for squeezing over.

Nutrition per serving
Kcals 463 • fat 24g • saturates 4g • carbs 33g • sugars 10g • fibre 4g • protein 31g • salt 0.32g

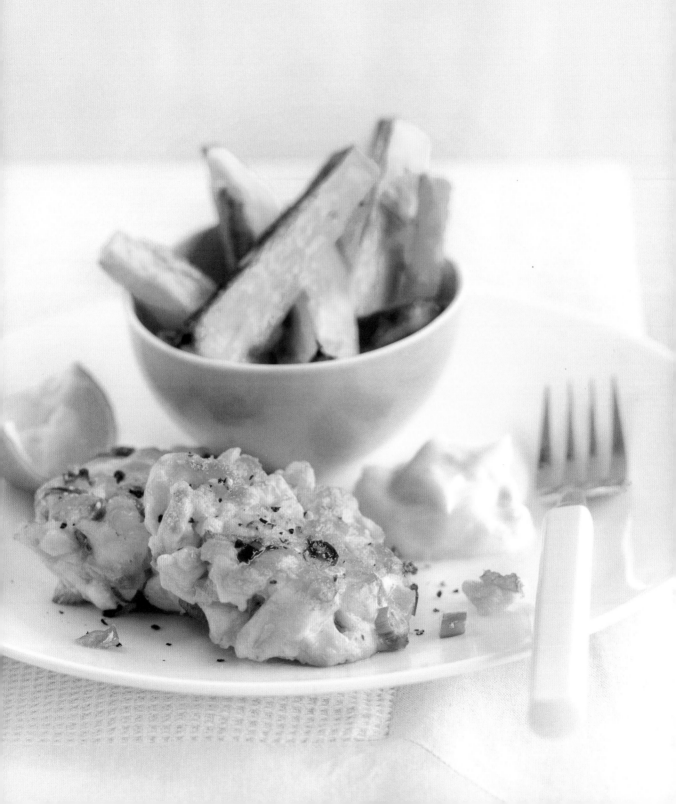

Pesto & olive crusted fish

A great way to pep up fish for a healthy, quick, midweek meal.

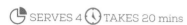 SERVES 4 ⏱ TAKES 20 mins

- 2 tbsp pesto
- finely grated zest 1 lemon
- 10 green olives, pitted and roughly chopped
- 85g fresh breadcrumbs
- 4 white fish fillets, such as cod or haddock

1 Heat oven to 200C/fan 180C/gas 6. Mix the pesto, lemon zest and olives together, then stir in the breadcrumbs.
2 Lay the fish fillets on a baking tray, skin-side down, then press the crumbs over the surface of each piece. Bake in the oven for 10–12 mins until the fish is cooked through and the crust is crisp and brown.

Nutrition per serving
Kcals 219 • fat 4g • saturates 1g • carbs 17g • sugars 1g • fibre 1g • protein 30g • Salt 1.14g

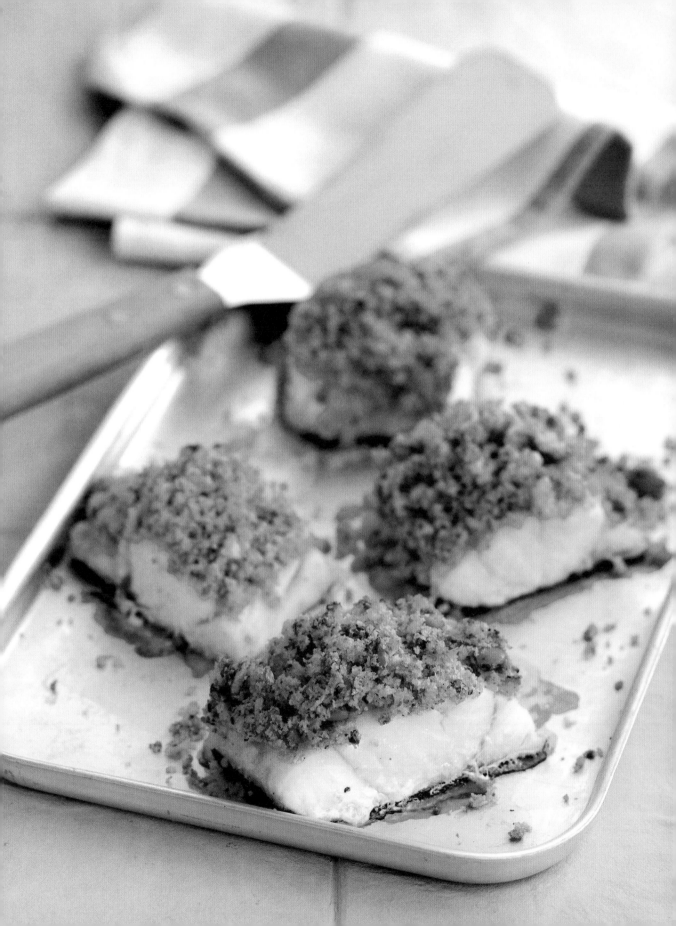

Fish finger tacos

Knock up this quick party snack using fish fingers, corn shells and a fennel coleslaw.

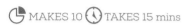 MAKES 10 TAKES 15 mins

- pack of 20 fish fingers
- 10 taco shells
- 300g tub ready-made coleslaw
- 1 fennel bulb, quartered and finely sliced
- zest and juice 1 lemon, plus wedges and extra zest to serve

1 Cook the fish fingers and warm the tacos following pack instructions. Meanwhile, mix the coleslaw with the fennel, lemon zest and juice, and some black pepper.
2 Divide the coleslaw and fish fingers among the warm tacos, sprinkle over the extra lemon zest and serve immediately with the lemon wedges.

Nutrition per taco
Kcals 255 • fat 16g • saturates 4g • carbs 18g • sugars 2g • fibre 3g • protein 9g • salt 0.8g

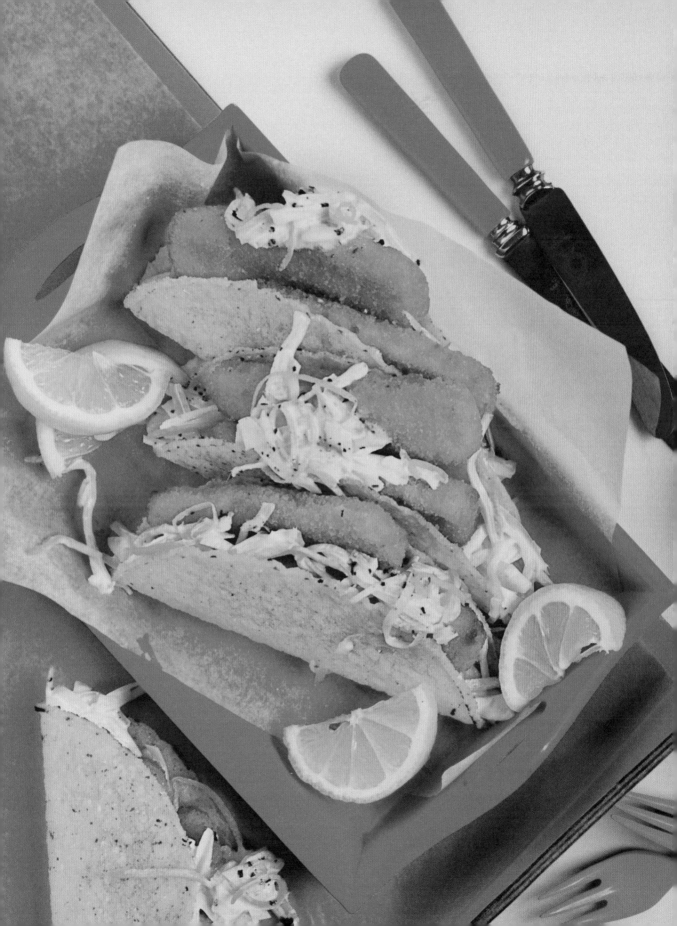

Seared seafood with bisque

Rustle up a luxurious, romantic (and speedy!) starter for 2 with fresh scallops, prawns and hot chilli.

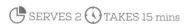 SERVES 2 ⏲ TAKES 15 mins

- 400g can lobster bisque
- 2 tbsp single cream, plus a little extra for drizzling
- 300g frozen seafood, we used a mixture of prawns and scallops, defrosted
- drizzle olive oil
- small handful coriander, leaves picked
- ½ red chilli, sliced

1 Heat the lobster bisque in a small pan until bubbling. Add the cream, reduce the heat and keep warm while you cook the seafood.

2 Season the seafood. Heat the oil in a frying pan. Add the seafood and cook for 1 min on each side until the prawns are pink and the scallops are cooked and starting to brown, but still have a little bounce.

3 To serve, pile the prawns and scallops into the centre of 2 shallow soup bowls, pour around the spicy bisque, scatter with a few coriander leaves, chilli slices and a drizzle of cream. Serve with toasted bread.

Nutrition per serving
Kcals 332 • fat 16g • saturates 9g • carbs 12g • sugars 5g • fibre 1g • protein 31g • salt 3.1g

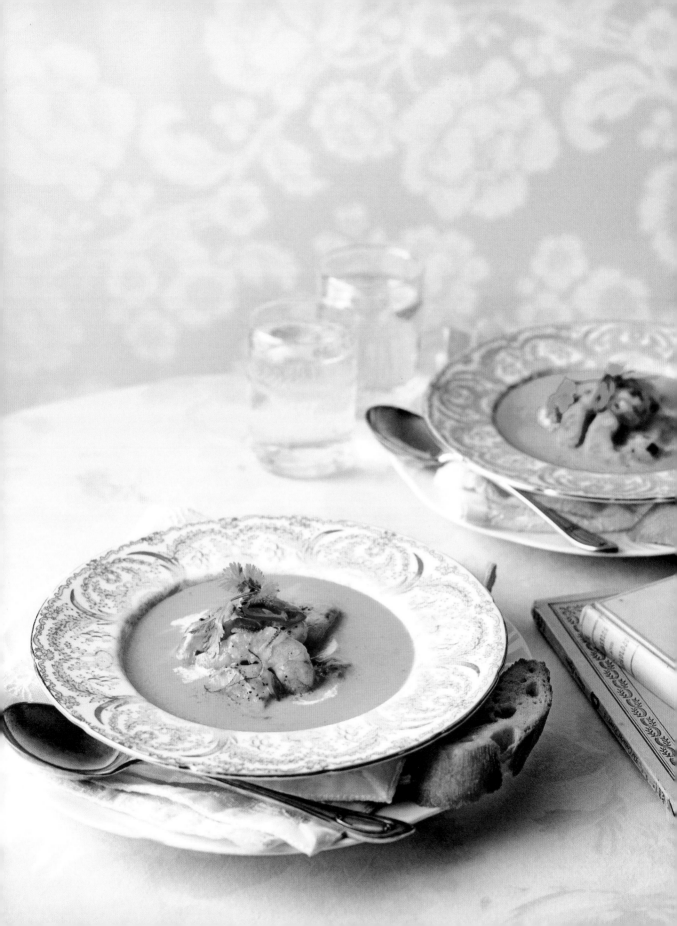

Mussels, white wine & parsley

British mussels are cheap, sustainable and surprisingly simple to cook.

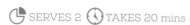 SERVES 2 TAKES 20 mins

- 1kg mussels, in shells
- small glass white wine
- 1 shallot, finely chopped
- chopped parsley, to serve

1 Tip the mussels into the sink or a large bowl of cold water. Swish them around with your hands to wash them thoroughly. Use a small sharp knife to scrape off any barnacles attached to the shells. Discard any mussels with broken shells.

2 Pull off the beards using the knife to help you – they just need a good tug. The beard is the brown wispy bit hanging out of the join in the shells. Not all mussels will have beards. If any mussels are open, tap them sharply against the side of the sink, worktop or with a knife. If they don't close, discard them – they are dead and not edible.

3 Rinse the mussels again in fresh cold water to remove any bits of shell or barnacle, and drain in a colander. Tip the mussels into a large pan, then add the wine and chopped shallot. The pan should not be more than half full – the mussels need plenty of space to move around so that they cook thoroughly.

4 Set the pan over a high heat and cover tightly with a lid. When the pan starts to steam, cook the mussels for 3–4 mins, shaking the pan from time to time to ensure they cook evenly. They are cooked when the shells have opened. Mussels that have not opened are fine to eat if they can be easily opened.

5 Remove the pan from the heat to stop the mussels cooking any further. Sprinkle with chopped parsley, then spoon them into warmed bowls and pour over the pan juices.

Nutrition per serving
Kcals 179 • fat 3g • saturates 1g • carbs 2g • sugars 2g • fibre 0g • protein 25g • salt 1.4g

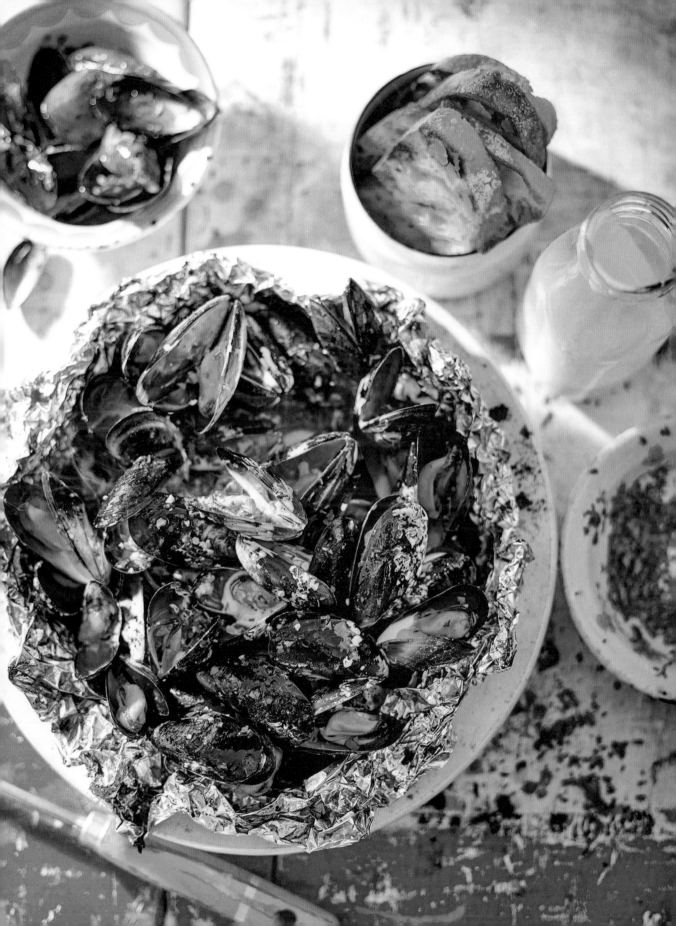

Citrus salmon salad

Zingy grapefruit, peppery watercress and crumbly feta take this simple salmon salad from nought to tasty in less than 10 minutes.

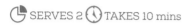 SERVES 2 ⏱ TAKES 10 mins

- 2 salmon fillets
- 1 large grapefruit
- 2 tbsp extra virgin olive oil
- 100g bag watercress
- ½ pack feta

1 Heat oven to 200C/180C fan/ gas 6 and roast the salmon for 8 mins. Meanwhile, segment the grapefruit and mix the juices with the extra virgin olive oil to make a dressing.
2 Toss the watercress with the grapefruit segments, the dressing and feta, and serve with the salmon, flaked into large pieces.

Nutrition per serving
Kcals 570 • fat 43g • saturates 12g • carbs 6g • sugars 6g • fibre 3g • protein 39g • salt 1.5g

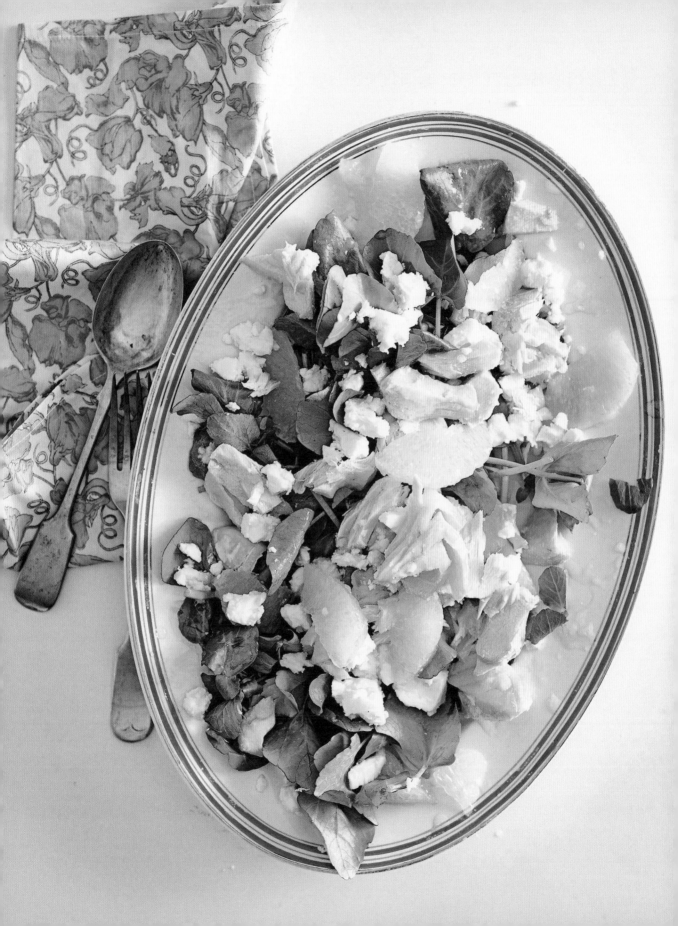

Warm tuna & lentil Niçoise salad

The simplest of salads that's 2 of your 5-a-day. This hearty lentil lunch will keep you going 'til dinner.

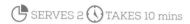 SERVES 2 TAKES 10 mins

- 2 medium eggs
- 1 pouch Puy lentils
- 1 pack mixed olive and veg antipasti
- 160g can or jar tuna in olive oil
- handful chopped parsley, optional

1 Cook the eggs in a pan of boiling water for 7 mins, then set aside in cold water. Tip the lentils into a saucepan and gently warm. Stir through the mixed antipasti in their oil, along with the tuna in large flakes. Season to taste. Gently peel the eggs and slice them in half. Spoon the warm lentils into bowls and top each one with the halved eggs and black pepper.

Nutrition per serving
Kcals 554 • fat 29g • saturates 5g • carbs 31g • sugars 3g • fibre 11g • protein 36g • salt 4.8g

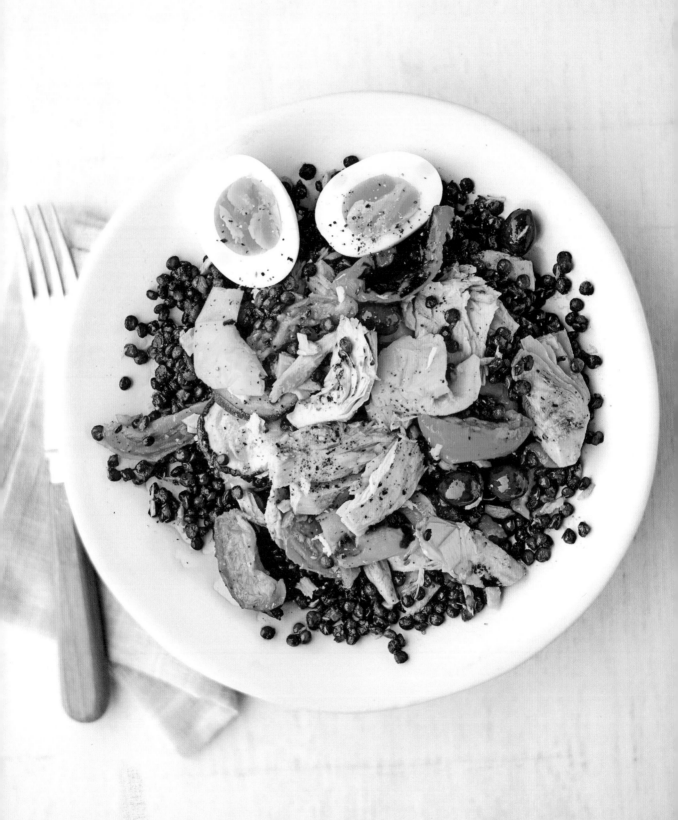

Baked cod with goat's cheese

Make a quick and easy, gluten-free, low-calorie lunch. The lean white fish is also a good source of protein and spinach contains vitamin K for bone health.

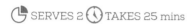 SERVES 2 　 TAKES 25 mins

- 1 tsp rapeseed oil
- 200g spinach
- 2 x 125g skinless cod fillets
- 25g soft goat's cheese
- 2 tomatoes, each sliced into 3
- a few thyme leaves

1 Heat oven to 200C/180C fan/gas 6. Heat the oil in a non-stick pan, tip in the spinach and stir until wilted. Spoon into the base of 2 gratin dishes, then top with the cod and season well.
2 Spread over some of the goat's cheese and arrange the tomatoes on top. Snip over a few thyme leaves, then bake for 10 mins until the fish flakes easily when tested. Serve in the dishes.

Nutrition per serving
Kcals 200 • fat 8g • saturates 2g • carbs 3g • sugars 3g • fibre 2g • protein 26g • salt 0.5g

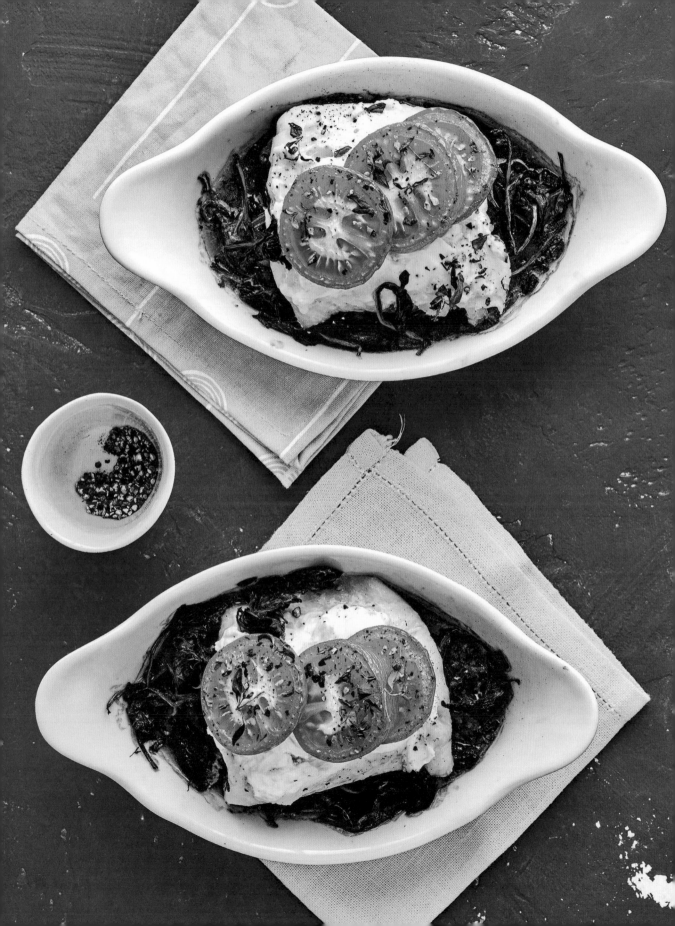

Saucy prawns

This satisfying, storecupboard meal-for-one will be on the table in just 20 minutes.

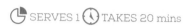 SERVES 1 TAKES 20 mins

- 1 garlic clove, crushed
- juice ½ lemon, plus wedges to serve
- 1 tbsp low sugar and salt ketchup
- 100ml chicken stock (from a cube is fine)
- 100g large cooked prawns

1 Heat the garlic, lemon juice, ketchup and stock together in a frying pan. Simmer until syrupy and thickened.
2 Add the prawns and some seasoning, then heat through. Serve with broccoli, steamed rice and lemon wedges.

Nutrition per serving
Kcals 127 • fat 1g • saturates 0g • carbs 4g • sugars 3g • fibre 1g • protein 26g • salt 2.3g

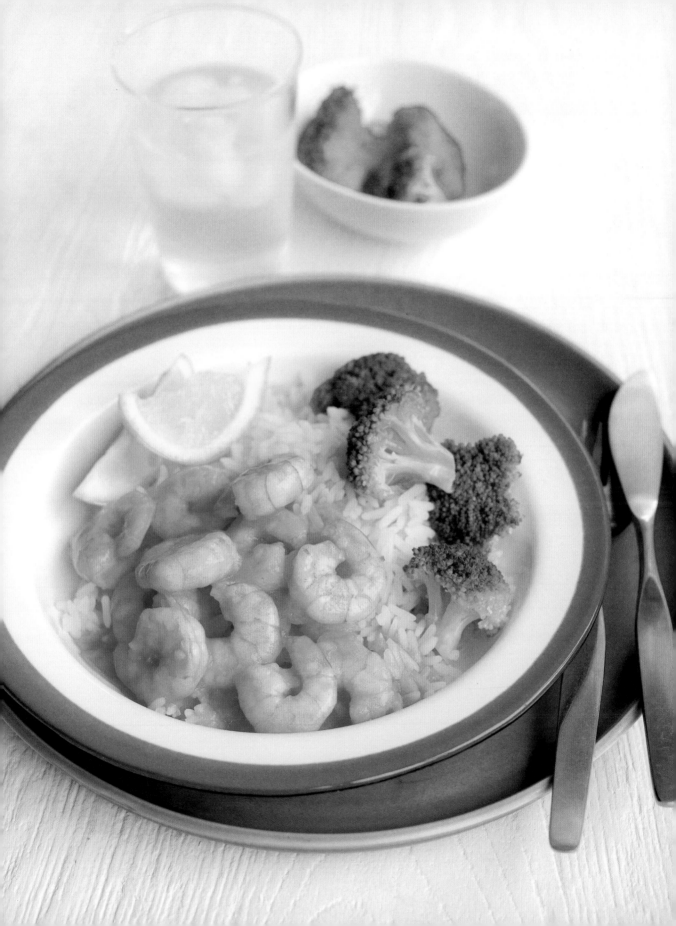

Creamy salmon & chive bows

Five ingredients is all you'll need for this fresh and light pasta dish of gravadlax and cream cheese.

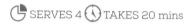 SERVES 4 TAKES 20 mins

- 350g farfalle
- 200g tub light soft cheese
- squeeze lemon juice
- 145g pack gravadlax, torn into pieces, or smoked salmon trimmings
- bunch chives, snipped

1 Cook the pasta following pack instructions. Once it's cooked, drain, reserving some of the water, and tip it back into the pan. Add the soft cheese, lemon juice and gravadlax or smoked salmon with some pepper and mix well. Add a little of the pasta water to help form a creamy sauce, and heat through.

2 Add most of the chives, stir, and divide the pasta mixture among bowls. Serve with the remaining chives scattered on top.

Nutrition per serving
Kcals 436 • fat 7g • saturates 3g • carbs 66g • sugars 4g • fibre 2g • protein 28g • salt 2.3g

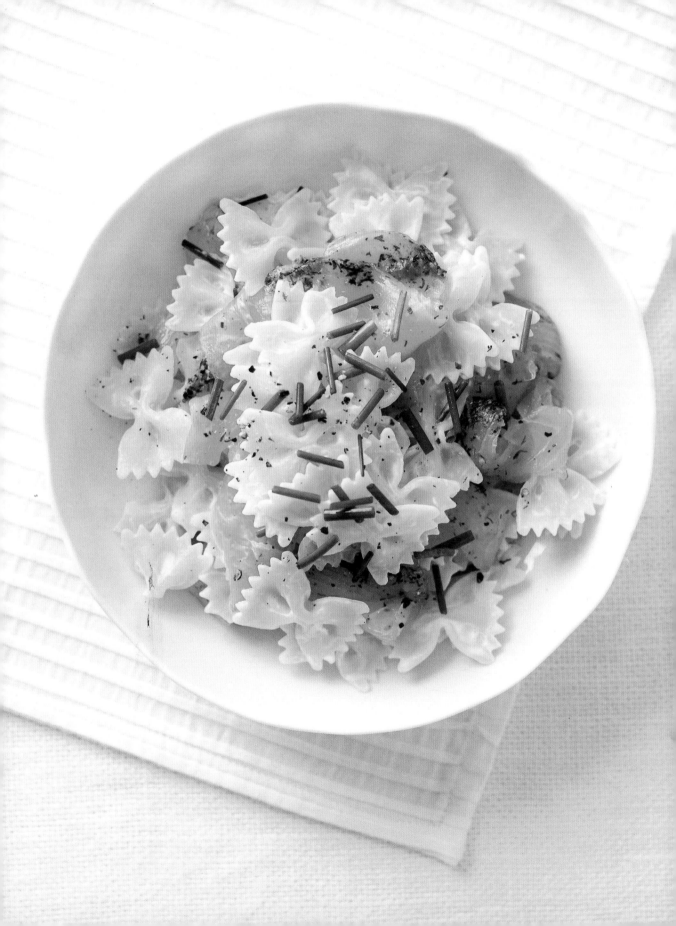

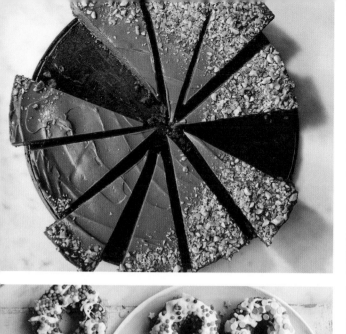
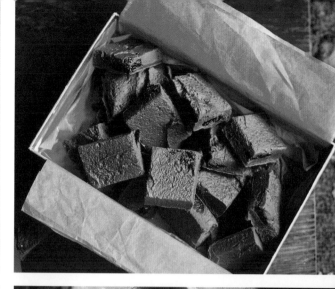
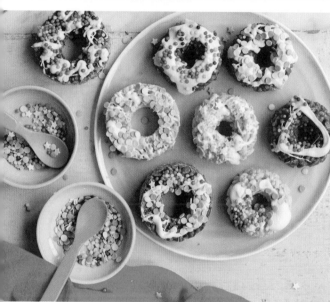
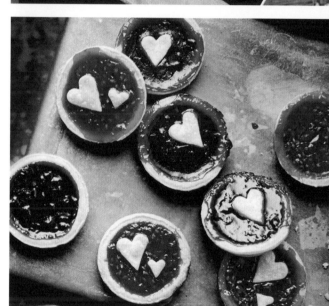
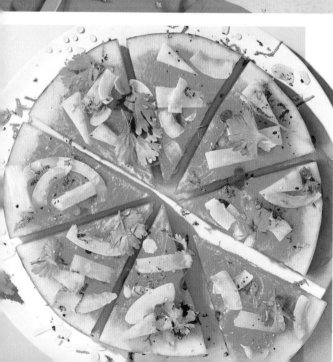
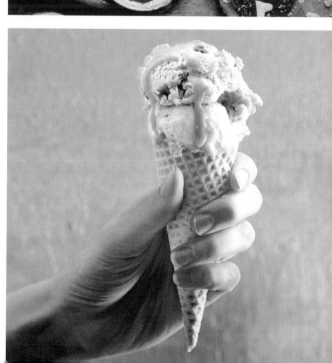

CHAPTER 7: DESSERTS & BAKING

Forget the long ingredients lists and challenging methods, these recipes will amaze you with their ease and speed. You'll wonder why you ever slaved over a complicated dessert once you've tried a handful of these recipes, all written with the busy cook in mind. This chapter also includes savoury bakes and bread – baking your own will save you money and is so satisfying. The Easy lentil pastries are perfect for a picnic, and the Fast truffle fudge makes the perfect gift at Christmas. Try the Dark chocolate & cherry bars if you want to impress – they won't last long.

Chocolate hazelnut ice cream cheesecake

No one will guess that this easy, rich and creamy no-cook, make-ahead cheesecake uses only 4 ingredients – ideal for a dinner party.

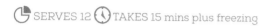 SERVES 12 TAKES 15 mins plus freezing

- 200g honey nut cornflakes
- 2 x 400g jars chocolate hazelnut spread
- 2 x 180g tubs full-fat cream cheese
- 1 tbsp roasted and chopped hazelnuts

1 Put the cornflakes and ½ a jar of chocolate hazelnut spread in a bowl and beat to combine – don't worry about breaking up the cornflakes. Press the mix into the base of a 23cm springform tin.

2 In a separate bowl, beat the cream cheese until smooth, then fold in the remaining chocolate hazelnut spread. Smooth onto the cornflake base, wrap tightly in cling film and freeze overnight.

3 Remove from the freezer 30 mins before serving, or until you can cut it easily with a sharp knife. Serve in slices with hazelnuts sprinkled over. Will keep in the freezer for up to 1 month.

Nutrition per serving
Kcals 542 · fat 33g · saturates 15g · carbs 50g · sugars 42g · fibre 3g · protein 8g · salt 0.5g

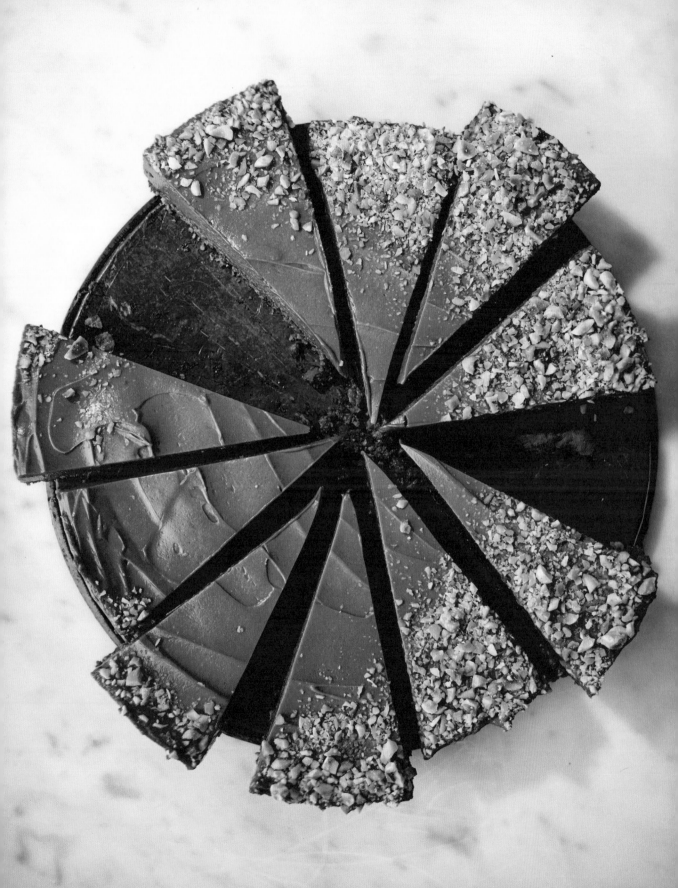

Buttermilk caramel puddings

A foolproof make-ahead spin on a crème caramel, using just 5 ingredients. The perfect winter dinner party dessert for those with a sweet tooth.

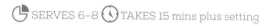 SERVES 6–8   TAKES 15 mins plus setting

- 350g white caster sugar
- 3 sheets leaf gelatine
- 600ml double cream
- 1 vanilla pod, split and seeds scraped out
- 284ml pot buttermilk

1 You'll need 6–8 dariole moulds or small individual pudding basins. Tip 150g of the sugar into a shallow pan and place over a medium heat. Cook the sugar until dissolved and turning to a light amber caramel. While it is still hot, carefully pour the caramel over the base of the moulds, tipping them around so some caramel also sticks to the sides. Set aside.

2 Soak the gelatine in very cold water for about 10 mins to soften. Tip the cream, remaining sugar and the vanilla pod and seeds into a saucepan. Place on the heat, stirring to combine and dissolve the sugar. Bring to a simmer, stirring occasionally, then remove from the heat. Add the drained, squeezed gelatine leaves and stir to dissolve, then leave to cool. When tepid, remove and squeeze out the vanilla pod, stir in the buttermilk, then strain everything into a jug. Share the mixture among the moulds, then place in the fridge for at least a couple of hours, or preferably overnight to set. Can be made up to 3 days ahead.

3 To serve, dip the bases of the moulds briefly into very hot water until the fillings just come away from the sides. When you are confident that it will turn out, place a serving plate over the mould and carefully turn, allowing the contents to drop out onto the plate, scooping out any caramel sauce left in the mould and drizzling over the puddings. Serve immediately.

Nutrition per serving (8)
Kcals 562 • fat 40g • saturates 25g • carbs 47g • sugars 47g • fibre 0g • protein 3g • salt 0.1g

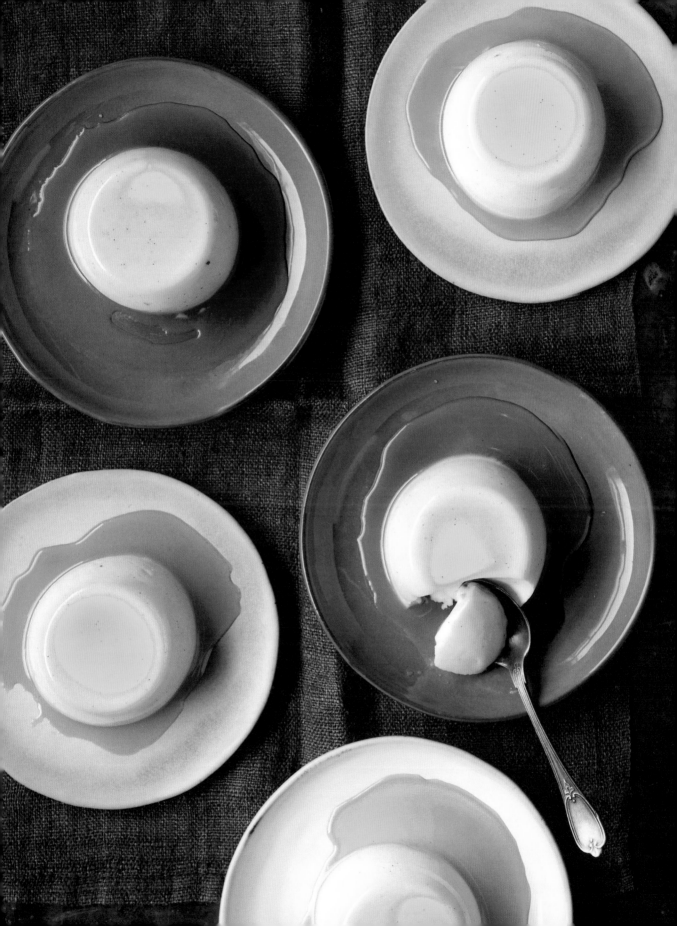

Coconut, caramel & pecan dairy-free ice cream

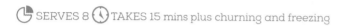

Catering for a dairy-free diet doesn't need to mean missing out on dessert. Enjoy this easy, creamy coconut, caramel and pecan ice cream as a treat.

SERVES 8 ⏱ TAKES 15 mins plus churning and freezing

- 2 x 400ml cans full-fat coconut milk
- 3 egg yolks
- 4 tbsp coconut sugar, or caster sugar
- dash vanilla extract
- 50g pecans, toasted and roughly chopped

1 Whisk the coconut milk until smooth. Measure 600ml into a saucepan and heat until just steaming. Meanwhile whisk the egg yolks with 3 tbsp sugar and the vanilla. Slowly pour the hot milk onto the yolks, whisking constantly. Wipe the pan clean, pour in the coconut and egg mixture, then cook over a medium heat, stirring for 5–6 mins until you have a thin custard. Strain and leave to cool completely, then churn in an ice cream maker.

2 To make the caramel, put the remaining coconut milk and sugar in a saucepan with a pinch of salt. Boil for 3 mins until it has the consistency of double cream. Cool, then swirl the caramel and pecans through the ice cream mix, cover the surface with cling film and freeze.

Nutrition per serving (8)
Kcals 275 • fat 23g • saturates 16g • carbs 13g • sugars 11g • fibre 1g • protein 3g • salt 0.01g

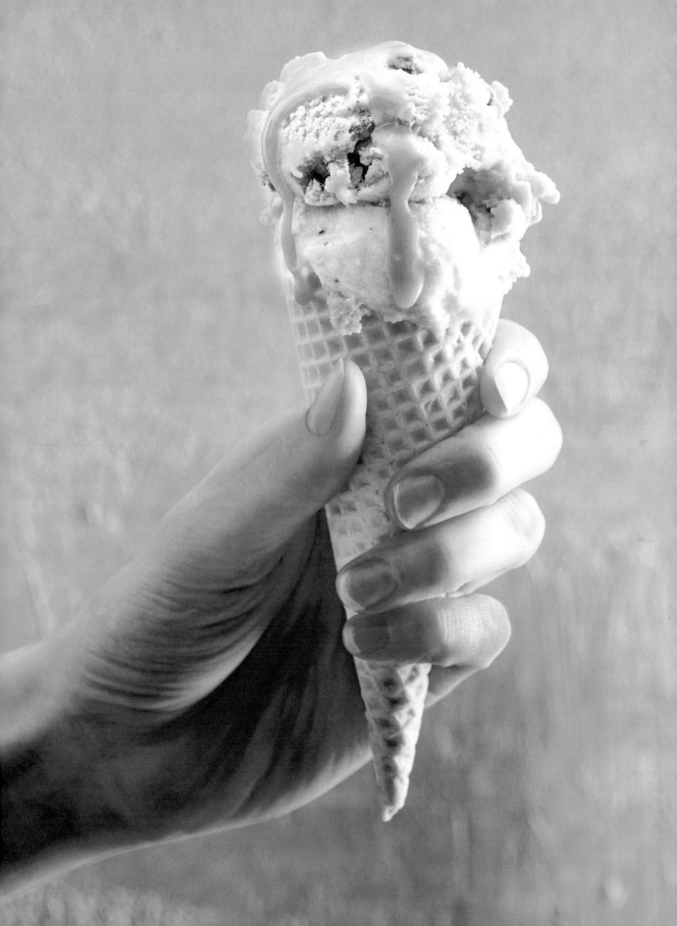

Giant mint choc ice

This ice cream and mint chocolate block takes just a handful of ingredients but is sure to impress. Ideal for feeding a crowd with a sweet tooth, simply slice and serve.

SERVES 6 · TAKES 25 mins plus freezing

- 2 tbsp vegetable oil, plus extra for the tin
- 200g dark chocolate
- 500ml good-quality vanilla ice cream
- 8 chocolate digestives or wafers
- 250g chocolate mint thins (around 24 individual chocolates)

1 Brush a 450g loaf tin with oil. As neatly as you can, line the bottom and sides of the tin with 2 strips of baking parchment. Melt 100g of the chocolate in the microwave with 1 tbsp vegetable oil on high in 30-sec bursts until smooth and glossy, then pour the melted chocolate into the loaf tin. Carefully spread the chocolate up the sides of the tin using a cutlery knife until they are all evenly coated. Put the tin in the freezer for 15 mins to set and take the ice cream out of the freezer to soften.

2 Take the tin out of the freezer and, working as quickly as you can, spread a quarter of the ice cream onto the base, then top with a single layer of chocolate mint thins. Add another layer of ice cream, followed by a layer of biscuits and mint thins. Top with another layer of ice cream, then a single layer of mint thins, before sealing with the last of the ice cream. Put back in the freezer to harden for at least 2 hrs or overnight. Don't worry if your layers are a bit messy – once everything has set and you cut a slice, it will all look great.

3 Melt the remaining chocolate with the remaining oil, leave it to cool a little, then, working quickly, spoon blobs over the ice cream and smooth over with the back of the spoon to cover the base. Return to the freezer until set. About 10 mins before you want to serve it, invert the ice cream bar onto a plate and peel off the baking parchment. Cut into 6 slices using a hot, sharp knife.

Nutrition per serving
Kcals 695 · fat 41g · saturates 22g · carbs 70g · sugars 54g · fibre 5g · protein 8g · salt 0.3g

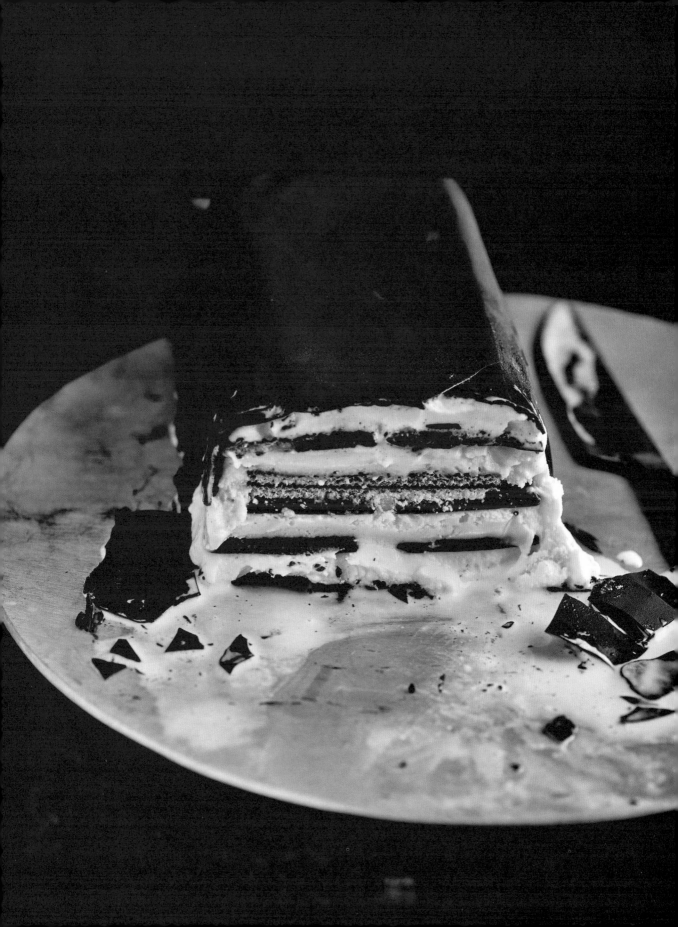

Lemon sorbet

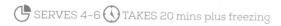

A simple and refreshing lemon sorbet with just 3 ingredients, serve as a light dessert or in between courses at a dinner party.

SERVES 4–6 ⏲ TAKES 20 mins plus freezing

- 250g white caster sugar
- juice of 2–3 lemons, plus a thick strip of lemon peel and lemon zest, to serve
- 2 tbsp vodka (optional)

1 Heat 250ml water, the sugar and the lemon peel in a small pan until the sugar has dissolved, then bring the mixture to the boil. Cook for 3 mins then turn off the heat and leave to cool. Pick out the lemon peel and discard. Measure out 100ml of lemon juice and add to the sugar mixture along with the vodka if using.
2 Pour into a freezer box and freeze for 1hr 30 mins then mix up with a whisk to break up and incorporate the ice crystals (which will be starting to form at the edges) before returning to the freezer.
3 Keep mixing the sorbet once an hour for 4 hours to break up the ice crystals. Stop mixing when firm but still scoopable, then store in the freezer for up to 1 month. Serve scoops of sorbet decorated with a few curls of lemon zest.

Nutrition per serving (6, including vodka)
Kcals 179 · fat 0g · saturates 0g · carbs 42g · sugars 42g · fibre 0g · protein 0g · salt 0g

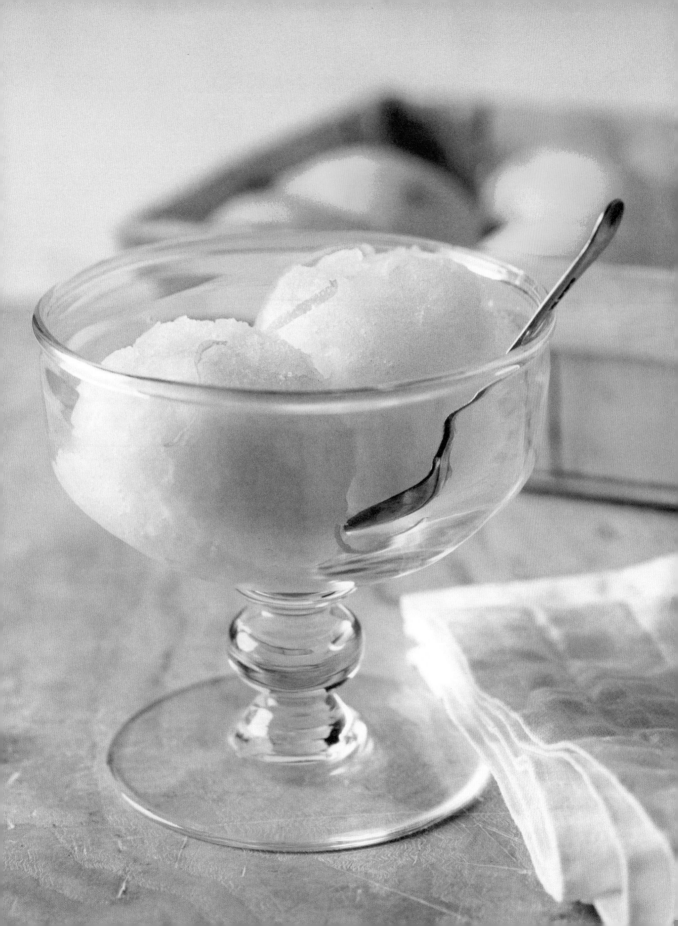

Watermelon pizza

Make this fun fruit 'pizza' as a side dish or a dessert at a picnic or barbecue. The watermelon, pineapple and coconut really sing summer. Drizzle with honey if you like it sweeter.

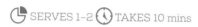 SERVES 1-2 🕐 TAKES 10 mins

- 1 slice watermelon
- 120g pineapple pieces
- a few coriander or Thai basil leaves
- 1–2 tsp toasted coconut flakes
- juice and zest ½ lime

1 Take 1 round slice of watermelon and cut into wedges, as you would a pizza, and lay them on a board. Scatter over the pineapple pieces, a few coriander or Thai basil leaves and the toasted coconut flakes. Drizzle the lime juice over the top. Sprinkle with freshly cracked black pepper and the lime zest.

Nutrition per serving
Kcals 112 • fat 2g • saturates 1g • carbs 22g • sugars 21g • fibre 2g • protein 1g • salt 0g

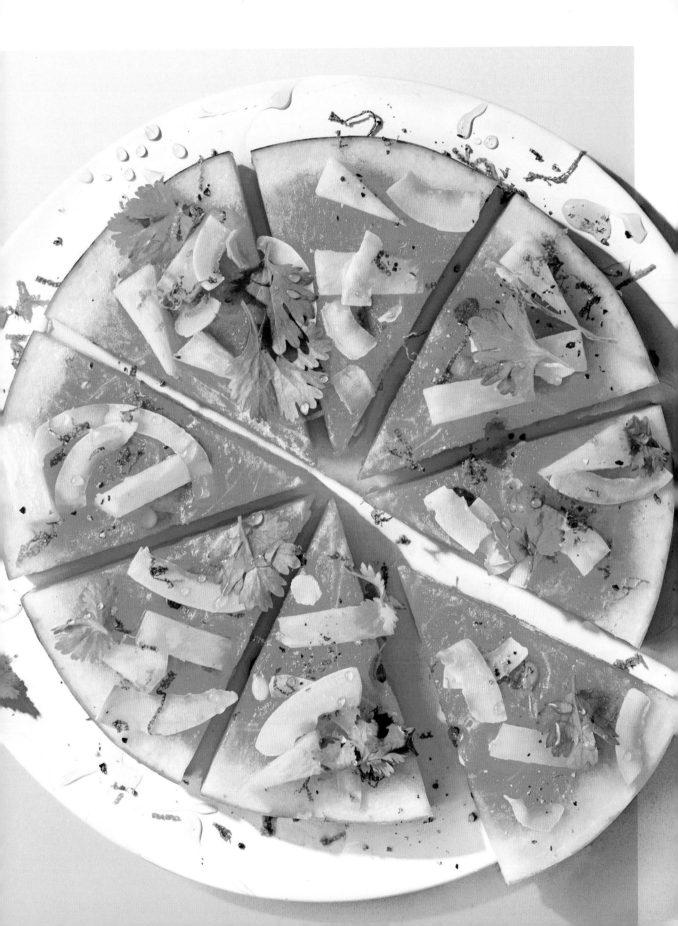

Fast truffle fudge

Make our truffle fudge in mere minutes and box it up with pretty tissue paper for the perfect homemade gift.

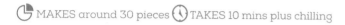 MAKES around 30 pieces TAKES 10 mins plus chilling

- 250g dark chocolate
- 25g butter
- 30g dried sour cherries
- 150g caramel or dulce de leche

1 Line an 18cm x 18cm brownie tin or similar-sized square food box with cling film. Put the dark chocolate and butter in a heatproof bowl and microwave until melted, stopping to stir the mixture every 30 seconds. Add in the sour cherries along with the caramel. Mix everything together then put into your prepared tin. Chill in the fridge until set (around 1 hr) then turn it out onto a board and remove the cling film. Chop into squares to serve.

Nutrition per serving
Kcals 71 • fat 5g • saturates 3g • carbs 6g • sugars 5g • fibre 1g • protein 1g • salt 0.04g

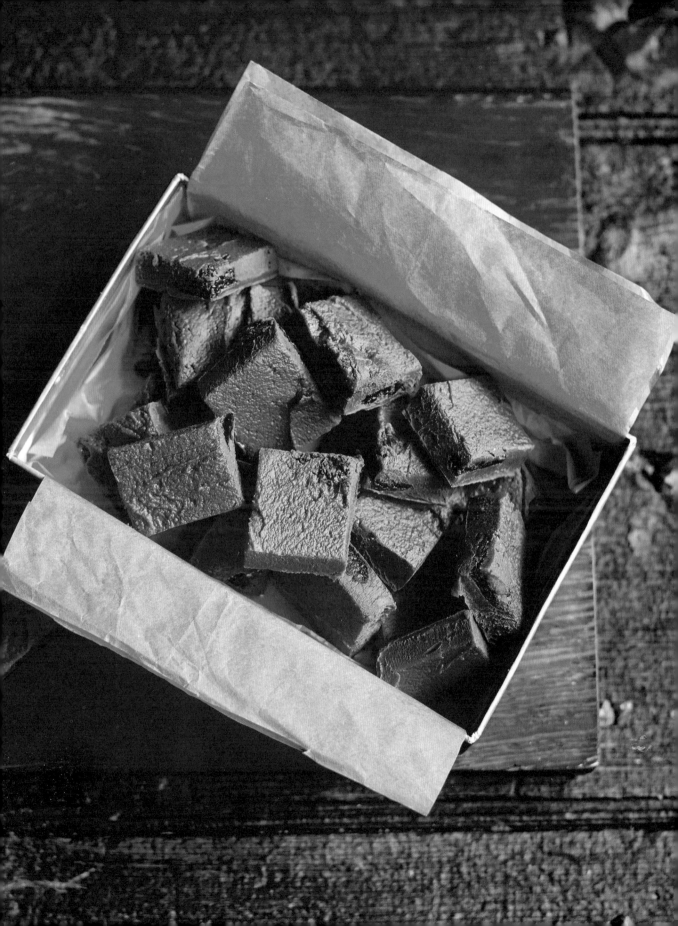

Swiss roll

The ultimate nostalgic treat, make your own Swiss roll with fruity strawberry jam filling. This easy dessert is great for entertaining.

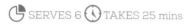 SERVES 6 TAKES 25 mins

- butter, for greasing
- 2 large eggs
- 50g caster sugar, plus extra 2 tbsp for dusting
- 50g self-raising flour, sieved
- 100g strawberry jam

1 Heat oven to 180C/160C fan/gas 4. Grease and line a 16cm x 28cm Swiss roll tin with baking parchment.
2 Beat the eggs and sugar together for 5 mins with an electric hand whisk until thick and pale. Gently fold in the flour in 2 batches using a large metal spoon. Pour the mixture into the tin and gently ease into the corners. Bake for 10–12 mins until golden and firm. Be careful not to overbake, or the sponge will break when rolled.
3 While the sponge is baking, sprinkle 2 tbsp sugar over a square of baking parchment. Warm the jam in the microwave for 20 secs.
4 Turn the baked sponge onto the sugared paper. Peel off the lining paper and spread the sponge with the warm jam. Roll up from the short edge using the paper to help you then cool on a wire rack.

Nutrition per serving
Kcals 162 • fat 3g • saturates 1g • carbs 31g • sugars 24g • fibre 0.3g • protein 4g • salt 0.2g

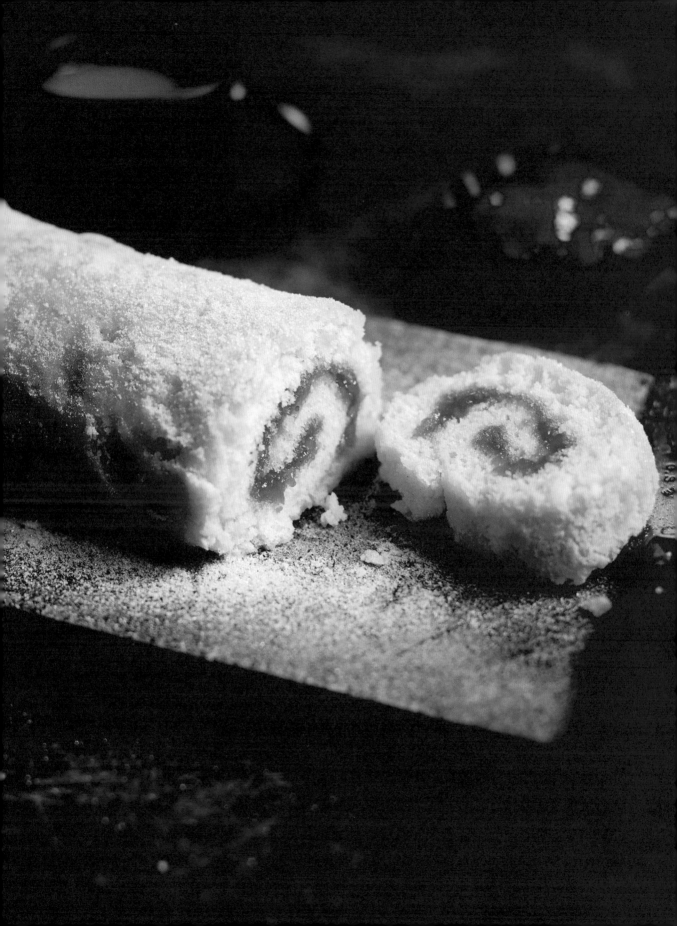

Yummy golden syrup flapjacks

Bake our 4-ingredient flapjacks – they're easy to make and ready in half-an-hour. Add chocolate drops, desiccated coconut or sultanas, if you like.

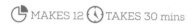 MAKES 12 TAKES 30 mins

- 250g jumbo porridge oats
- 125g butter, plus extra for the tin
- 125g light brown sugar
- 2–3 tbsp golden syrup (depending on how gooey you want it)

1 Heat oven to 200C/180C fan/gas 6. Put all the ingredients in a food processor and pulse until mixed, but be careful not to overmix otherwise the oats may lose their texture.
2 Lightly grease a 20cm x 20cm baking tin with butter and spoon in the mixture. Press into the corners with the back of a spoon so the mixture is flat and score into 12 squares. Bake for around 15 minutes until golden brown.

Nutrition per serving
Kcals 212 • fat 10g • saturates 6g • carbs 27g • sugars 13g • fibre 2g • protein 2g • salt 0.3g

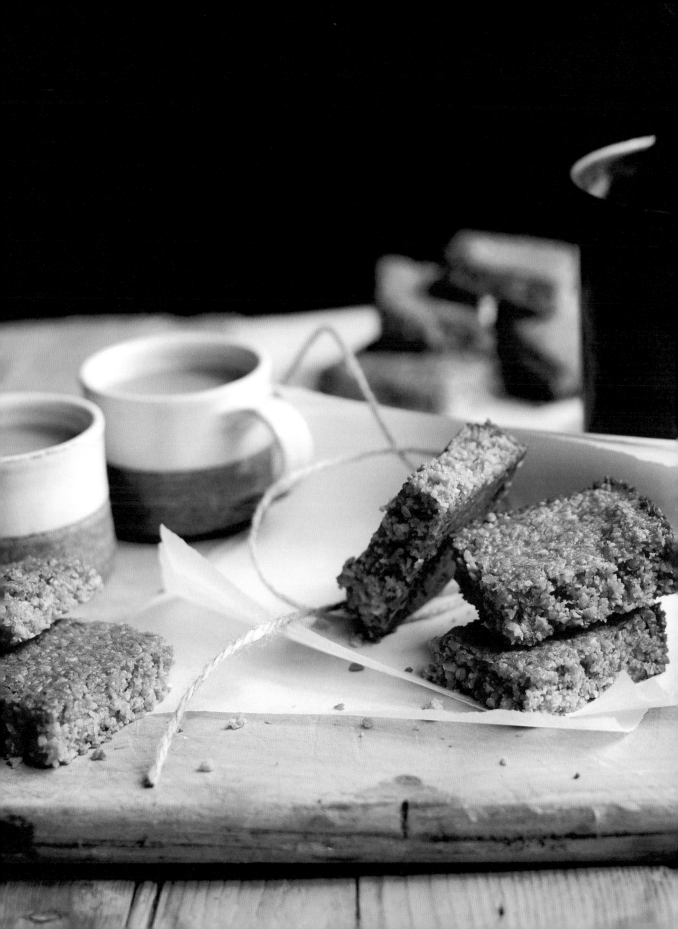

Rice pop doughnuts

These rice pop doughnuts are a fun activity for kids to get stuck into over the holidays. Just a few ingredients needed, no baking and plenty of sprinkles.

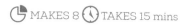 MAKES 8 TAKES 15 mins

- 200g dark, milk or white chocolate, chopped, plus extra white chocolate for decorating
- 25g butter, plus extra for the moulds
- 2 tbsp golden syrup
- 80g rice pops cereal
- sprinkles, for decorating

1 Line an A4-sized baking tray with cling film, or butter a tray of doughnut moulds. Very gently melt the chocolate, butter and golden syrup together in a bowl set over a pan of simmering water, or in a microwave by heating it in short blasts and stirring between each blast.
2 Take the chocolate off the heat and mix into the rice pops, making sure they are all covered in the mixture.
3 Spoon the rice pops onto the lined baking tray and press the mixture down firmly so it fills any gaps, or divide the mixture among the moulds. Set the mixture aside somewhere cool to set hard.
4 Once set, if you used a tray, cut 8 doughnut shapes using a 9cm round cutter and a 2cm round cutter for the hole in the middle. Melt the white chocolate in the microwave and drizzle over the doughnuts, then top with the sprinkles to decorate.

Nutrition per doughnut
Kcals 278 • fat 14g • saturates 8g • carbs 34g • sugars 24g • fibre 1g • protein 3g • salt 0.4g

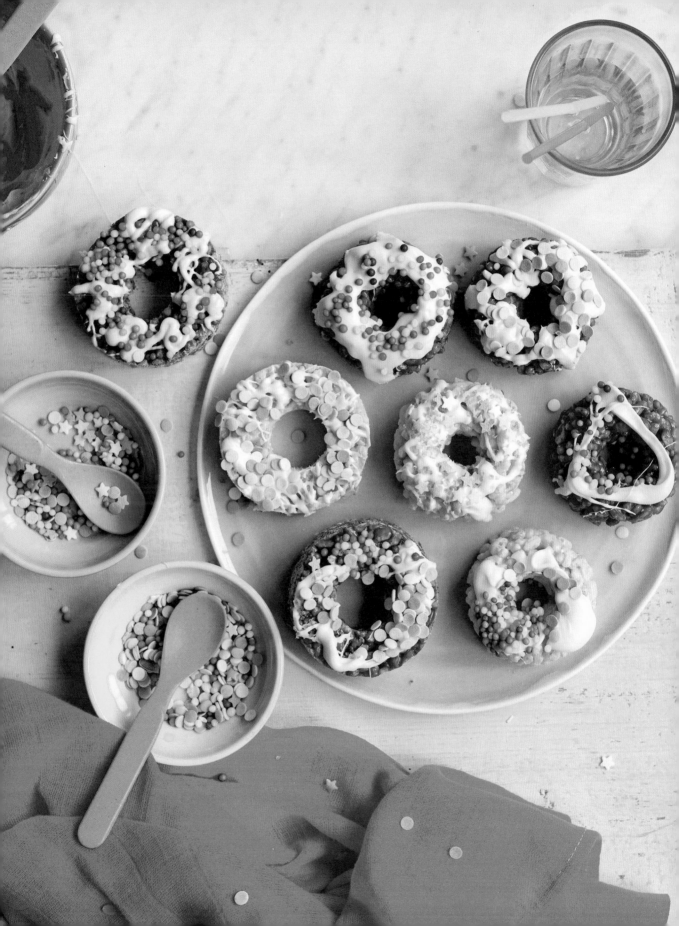

Really easy cinnamon rolls

Use ready-made croissant dough to make these easy cinnamon rolls. We've topped the rolls with a thick caramel, but you could use a thin white icing instead.

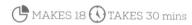 MAKES 18 ⏱ TAKES 30 mins

- 350g can ready-made croissant dough (we used Jus Rol)
- 30g unsalted butter, softened
- 2 tsp cinnamon
- 6 tbsp soft light brown sugar

1 Heat oven to 180C/160C fan/gas 4. Line a 23cm cake tin with a square of baking parchment so the corners stick up (this will help you to lift the rolls out).

2 Unroll the croissant dough from the can and lay it out on your work surface. Cut it into 3 sections along the dotted lines, but don't cut the diagonal line. Spread over a quarter of the butter.

3 Mix the cinnamon and sugar together. Using 1 square of dough at a time, sprinkle over 2–3 tsp of the sugar and roll up the dough. When you have 3 rolls, cut each one in ½ and then each ½ into 3. Arrange the rolls in the tin in 2 circles – you need to spread them well apart as they will rise and spread. Stick the end bits in among fatter pieces from the centre of the rolls so they cook evenly. Bake for 15 mins or until the rolls are risen and cooked through.

4 Meanwhile, heat the remaining sugar mix with the remaining butter until you have a thick caramel (don't worry if some of the butter separates out, it will soak into the dough). When the rolls are cooked, pour over the caramel. Leave to cool a little, then eat warm.

Nutrition per serving
Kcals 109 • fat 6g • saturates 3g • carbs 13g • sugars 8g • fibre 0g • protein 1g • salt 0.2g

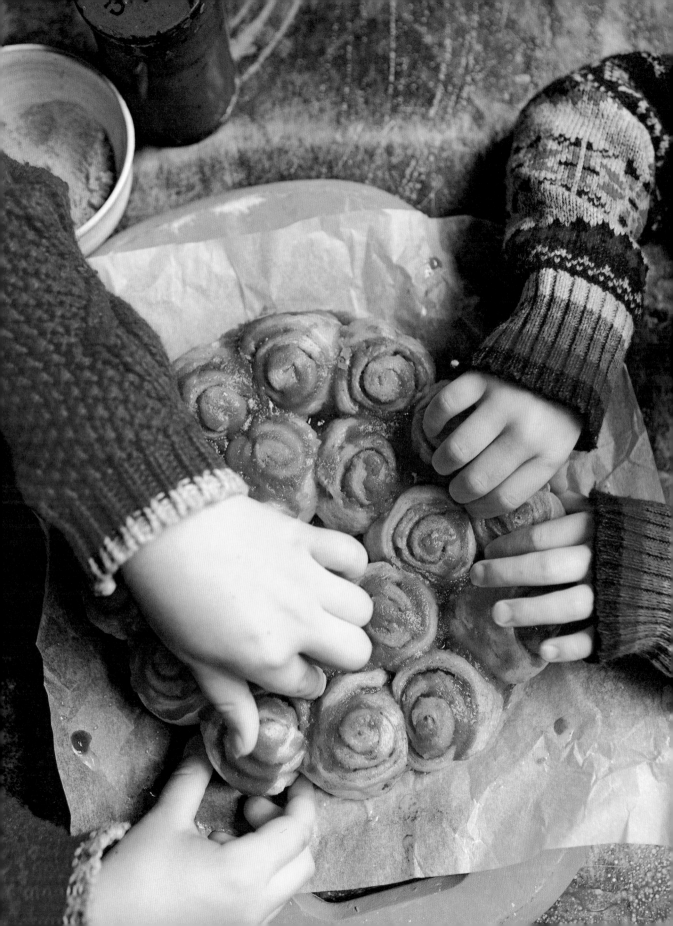

Dark chocolate & cherry bar

This impressive looking dessert is a chocolate lover's dream and no one will guess it uses just 4 ingredients.

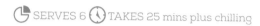 SERVES 6 ⏱ TAKES 25 mins plus chilling

- 80g amaretti biscuits, roughly crushed
- 400g good-quality (60%) dark chocolate, chopped
- 400ml double cream
- 390g jar cherries in kirsch

1 Line a 20cm square baking tin with a strip of baking parchment – leave an overhang as this will help lift everything out of the tin later. Scatter the amaretti biscuits over the base of the tin and set aside.

2 Tip the chocolate into a heatproof bowl and pour the cream into a saucepan. Bring the cream to the boil, then pour it over the chocolate and stir until completely melted. Pour the mixture over the biscuits, then tap the tin to even out. Cover with cling film and chill in the fridge for at least 4 hrs (or up to 2 days ahead).

3 While the chocolate is setting, drain the cherries over a small saucepan and set them aside. Simmer the juice from the jar for about 5 mins or until syrupy. This can be done a day ahead and both can be kept in the fridge.

4 To serve, use the parchment handles to lift everything out of the tin on to a board and, using a sharp knife dipped in hot water, cut into 6 neat bars. Using a pastry brush, paint a thick stripe of the kirsch syrup across each plate, then sit a chocolate bar across the stripe at an opposing angle. Top each bar with a line of cherries and serve with extra syrup on the side.

Nutrition per serving
Kcals 783 • fat 62g • saturates 37g • carbs 47g • sugars 35g • fibre 6g • protein 6g • salt 0.1g

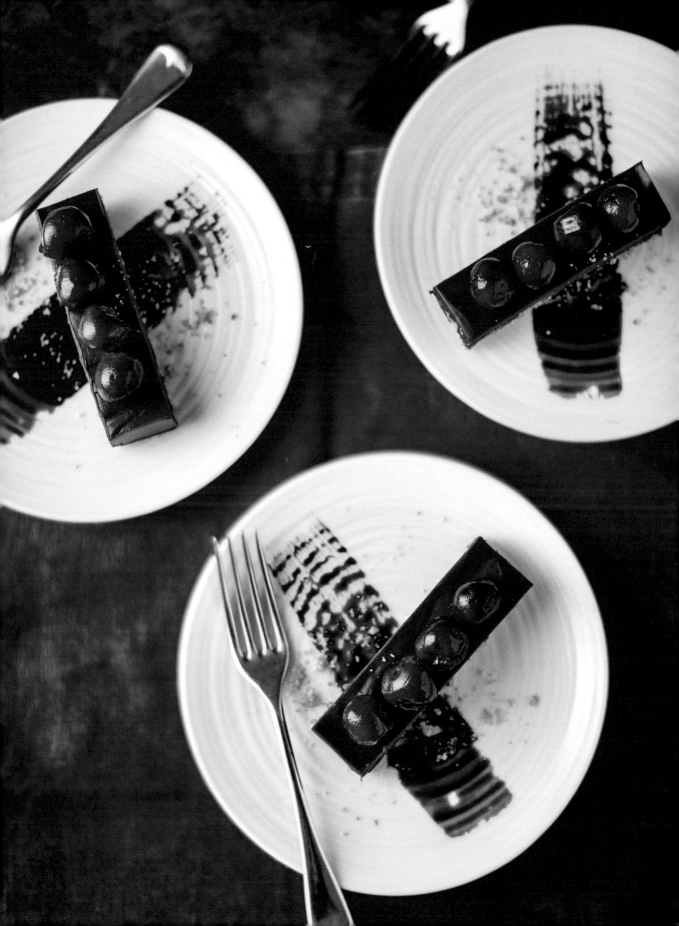

Peanut butter cookies

With just 4 ingredients, these simple peanut butter cookies will delight kids and grown-ups alike – and they're gluten-free, too.

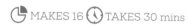 MAKES 16 TAKES 30 mins

- 200g peanut butter (crunchy or smooth is fine)
- 175g golden caster sugar
- ¼ tsp fine table salt
- 1 large egg

1 Heat oven to 180C/160C fan/gas 4 and line 2 large baking trays with baking parchment.
2 Measure the peanut butter and sugar into a bowl. Add the fine table salt and mix well with a wooden spoon. Add the egg and mix again until the mixture forms a dough.
3 Break off cherry tomato-sized chunks of dough and place, well spaced apart, on the trays. Press the cookies down with the back of a fork to squash them a little. The cookies can now be frozen for 2 months and cooked from frozen, adding an extra min or 2 to the cooking time.
4 Bake for 12 mins, until golden around the edges and paler in the centre. Cool on the trays for 10 mins, then transfer to a wire rack and cool completely. Store in a cookie jar for up to 3 days.

Nutrition per serving
Kcals 126 • fat 7g • saturates 2g • carbs 12g • sugars 11g • fibre 0.5g • protein 4g • salt 0.2g

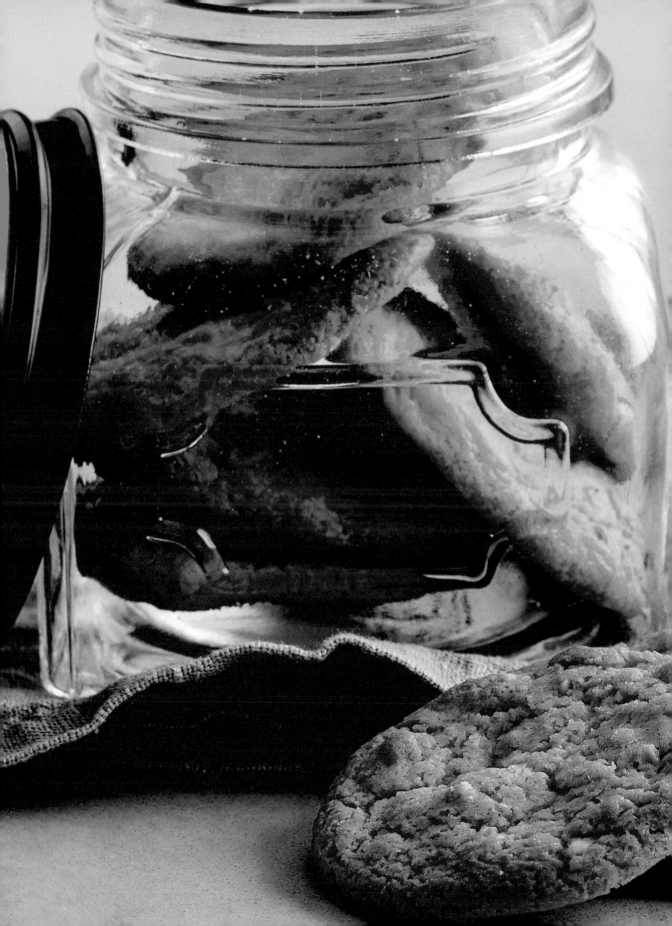

Simple iced biscuits

You can add some lemon zest or vanilla extract to these simple biscuits if you like.

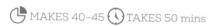 MAKES 40–45 🕐 TAKES 50 mins

- 200g unsalted butter, softened
- 200g golden caster sugar
- 1 large egg
- 400g plain flour, plus extra for dusting
- 8–12 x 19g coloured icing pens, or fondant icing sugar mixed with a little water and food colouring

1 Heat oven to 200C/180C fan/gas 6. Put the butter in a bowl and beat it using an electric whisk until soft and creamy. Beat in the sugar, then the egg and finally the flour to make a dough. If the dough feels a bit sticky, add a little more flour and knead it in.

2 Cut the dough into 6 pieces and roll out one at a time to about 5mm thickness on a floured surface. The easiest way to do this is to roll the mixture out on a baking mat. Cut out letter and number shapes (we used 7cm x 4cm cutters) and peel away the leftover dough at the edges. Re-roll any off-cuts and repeat.

3 Transfer the whole mat or the individual biscuits to 2 baking sheets (transfer them to baking parchment if not using a mat) and bake for 7–10 mins or until the edges are just brown. Leave to cool completely and repeat with the rest of the dough. You should be able to fit about 12 on each sheet. If you are using 2 sheets, then the one underneath will take a minute longer.

4 Ice the biscuits using the pens to make stripes or dots, or colour in the whole biscuit if you like. They will keep for 5 days in an airtight container.

Nutrition per biscuit
Kcals 86 • fat 4g • saturates 2g • carbs 11g • sugars 4g • fibre 0g • protein 1g • salt 0.2g

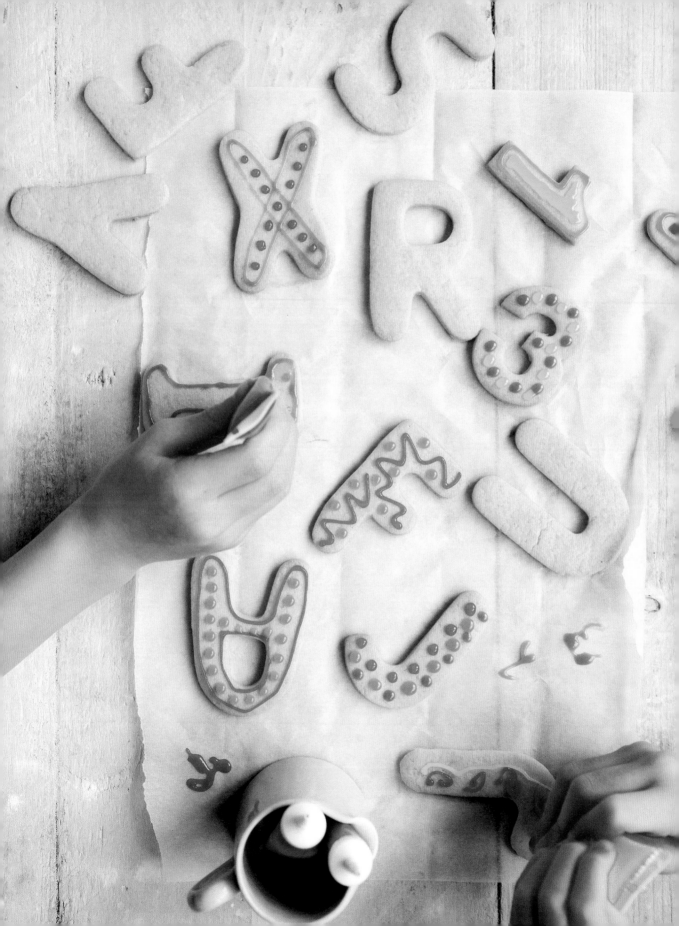

Shortbread

Bake these classic shortbread biscuits to wow a crowd. You only need 4 ingredients, but you can mix it up with lemon or orange zest, or try adding chopped pistachios.

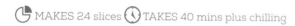 MAKES 24 slices TAKES 40 mins plus chilling

- 300g butter, softened
- 140g golden caster sugar, plus 4 tbsp
- 300g plain flour
- 140g rice flour

1 Place the butter and sugar in a food processor and whizz until smooth.
2 Tip in both the flours and a pinch of salt, then whizz until mixture comes together.
3 Using your hands, roughly spread the mixture out in a 20cm x 30cm x 4cm baking tray. Cover with cling film and smooth over until there are no wrinkles. Place in the fridge, uncooked, for at least 30 mins and up to 2 days.
4 Heat oven to 180C/160C fan/gas 4. Remove cling film, then lightly mark the shortbread all over with a fork.
5 Sprinkle with the remaining sugar, then bake for 20–25 mins.
6 Leave to cool in the tin, then cut into 24 thin slices. Shortbread will keep in an airtight container for up to 1 week.

Nutrition per slice
Kcals 188 • fat 11g • saturates 7g • carbs 23g • sugars 9g • fibre 0g • protein 2g • salt 0.2g

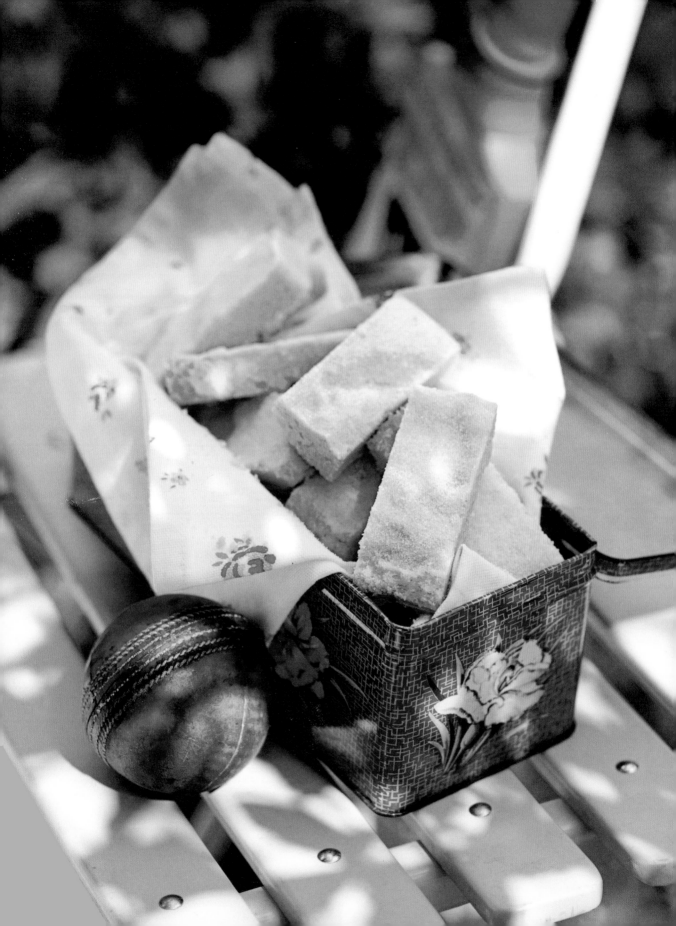

Jam tarts

Bake our easy jam tarts and they'll instantly become a family favourite – plus, you can make them in less than half-an-hour if you use ready-made pastry.

SERVES 12 TAKES 40 mins plus chilling

- 250g plain flour, plus extra for dusting
- 125g butter, chilled and diced, plus extra for the tin
- 1 medium egg
- 1 vanilla pod, seeds scraped (optional)
- 100g jam, fruit curd or marmalade of your choice

1 Put the flour, butter and a pinch of salt in a bowl and rub them together with your fingertips (or you can pulse these ingredients together in a food processor if you have one). When the mixture looks and feels like fresh breadcrumbs, stir in the egg and vanilla seeds, if using, with a cutlery knife. Add 1 tbsp cold water, then start to bring the dough together in one lump with your hands – try not to knead it too much. Add 1 more tbsp of water if it's not coming together, but try not to add more than that. Wrap in cling film and chill in the fridge for 30 mins.

2 Heat oven to 200C/180C fan/gas 6. Butter a 12-hole tart tin, then dust your work surface with flour. Unwrap and roll out the chilled pastry so it's about the thickness of a £1 coin, then use a straight or fluted round cutter to cut out 12 circles, big enough to line the holes in the tin. Dollop 1–2 tsp of your chosen filling into each one and, if you like, cut out little pastry hearts (perfect for Valentine's Day) and pop them on top.

3 Bake for 15–18 mins or until golden and the filling is starting to bubble a little. Leave to cool in the tin for a few mins then carefully transfer to a wire rack to cool completely.

Nutrition per serving
Kcals 183 • fat 9g • saturates 6g • carbs 22g • sugars 6g • fibre 1g • protein 3g • salt 0.2g

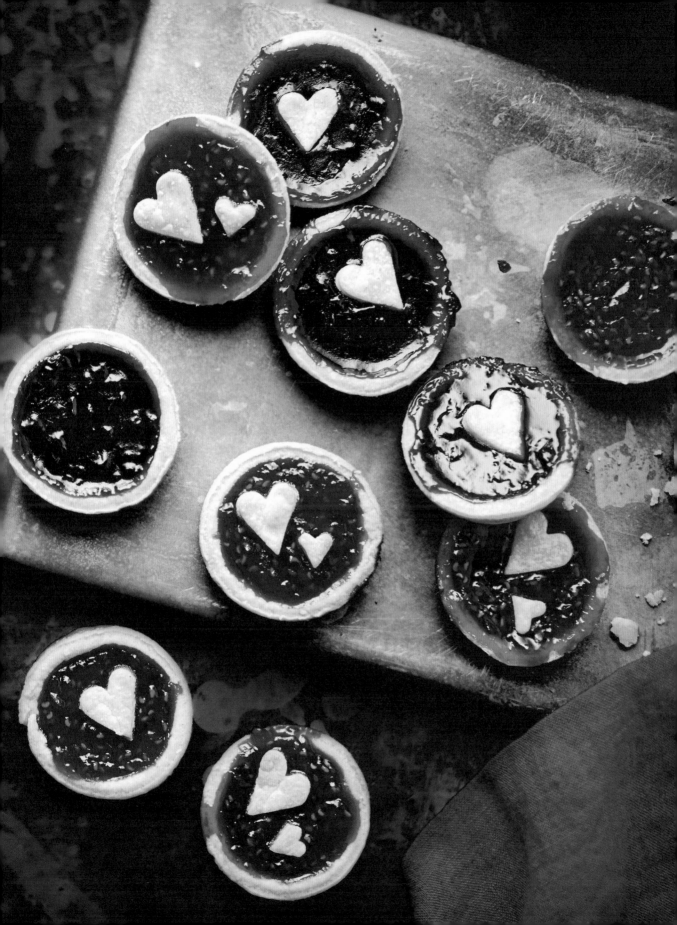

Easy lentil pastries

Make savoury bakes the easy way – our tasty pastry pockets filled with lentils and feta are ideal for a quick lunch, starter or snack.

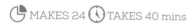 MAKES 24 ⏱ TAKES 40 mins

- 320g shortcrust pastry sheet
- 250g pouch Puy lentils
- 200g jar sundried tomatoes, drained and chopped
- 100g feta
- 1 egg

1 Heat oven to 200C/180C fan/gas 6. Unroll the pastry and cut into 24 squares. Mix the lentils, tomatoes and feta with some seasoning and divide among the pastry squares, leaving a border around the edge. Beat the egg and brush a little of it onto the edges of the pastry, then pinch together to seal in a cross shape at the top. Transfer the pastries to a large baking sheet, brush with the remaining beaten egg and bake for 20 mins until golden. Serve as a starter with dressed leaves.

Nutrition per serving
Kcals 353 • fat 22g • saturates 9g • carbs 26g • sugars 2g • fibre 4g • protein 9g • salt 1.3g

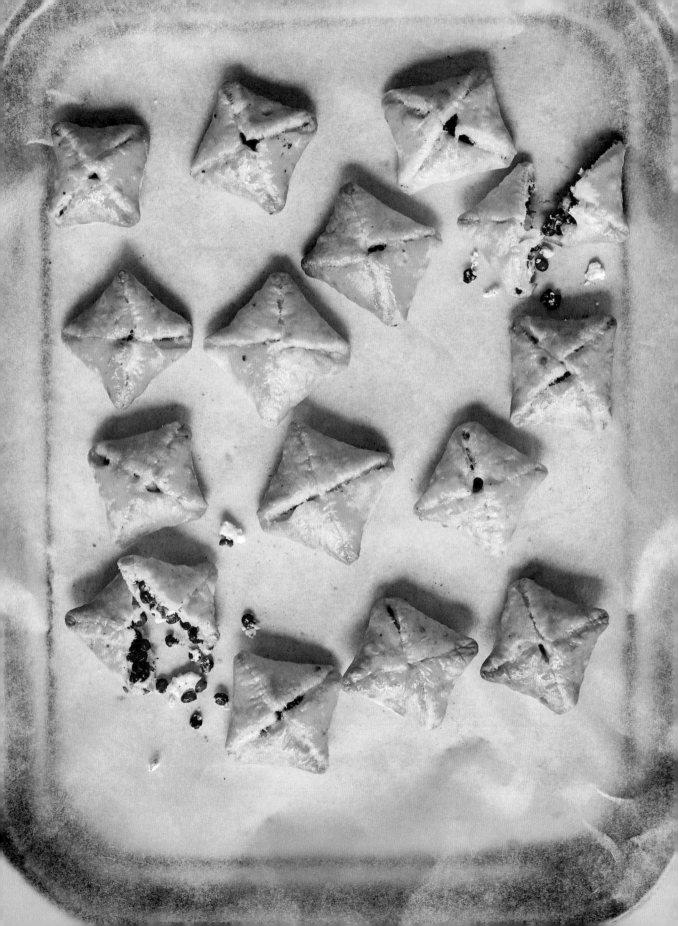

Wholemeal sourdough

Try making our easy sourdough loaf and fill your home with a gorgeous aroma as it bakes. You need to have a sourdough starter which you can make yourself.

 MAKES 1 loaf ⏱ TAKES 2 hrs plus rising (and 8 days for the starter)

TO MAKE THE SOURDOUGH STARTER
- 200g strong white flour
- 200g strong wholemeal flour

TO MAKE THE SOURDOUGH BREAD
- 450g strong white flour, plus extra for dusting
- 50g wholemeal flour
- 10g fine salt
- 100g sourdough starter (see above)

1 To make a sourdough starter: whisk 50g of the strong white flour and 50g of the strong wholemeal flour with 100ml slightly warm water until smooth. Transfer to a large jar or plastic container. Leave the lid ajar for 1 hr or so in a warm place, then seal and set aside for 24 hours. For the next 6 days, you will need to 'feed' it. Each day, tip away half the original starter, add an extra 25g of each flour and 50ml slightly warm water, and stir well. After a few days you should start to see bubbles on the surface, and it will smell yeasty. On day 7 the starter should be bubbly and smell much sweeter. It is now ready to be used.

2 To make the sourdough bread: tip both the flours, 325ml warm water, the salt and the starter into a bowl, or a mixer fitted with a dough hook. Stir with a wooden spoon, or on a slow setting in the mixer until combined – add extra flour if it's too sticky or a little warm water if it's dry. Tip onto a lightly floured surface and knead for 10 mins until soft and elastic – you should be able to stretch it without it tearing. If you're using a mixer, turn up the speed a little and mix for 5 mins.

3 Place the dough in a floured bowl and cover with cling film. Leave in a warm place to rise for 3 hrs. You may not see much movement, as sourdough takes much longer to rise.

4 Line a medium bowl with a clean tea towel and flour it really well or flour a proving basket. Tip the dough back onto your work surface and knead briefly to knock out any air bubbles. Shape the dough into a smooth ball and dust it with flour.

5 Place the dough, seam-side up, in the bowl or proving basket, and leave at room temperature for 3 hrs, or in the fridge overnight, until risen by about a quarter.

6 Place a large baking tray in the oven and heat to 230C/210C fan/gas 8. Fill a small roasting tin with water and place in the bottom of the oven to create steam. Remove the tray from the oven, sprinkle with flour, then tip the dough onto it.

7 Slash the top a few times with a sharp knife to make a pattern, then bake for 35–40 mins until golden brown. It should sound hollow when tapped on the bottom. Leave to cool on a wire rack before slicing.

Nutrition per serving
Kcals 245 • fat 1g • saturates 0g • carbs 48g • sugars 1g • fibre 2g • protein 8g • salt 0.4g

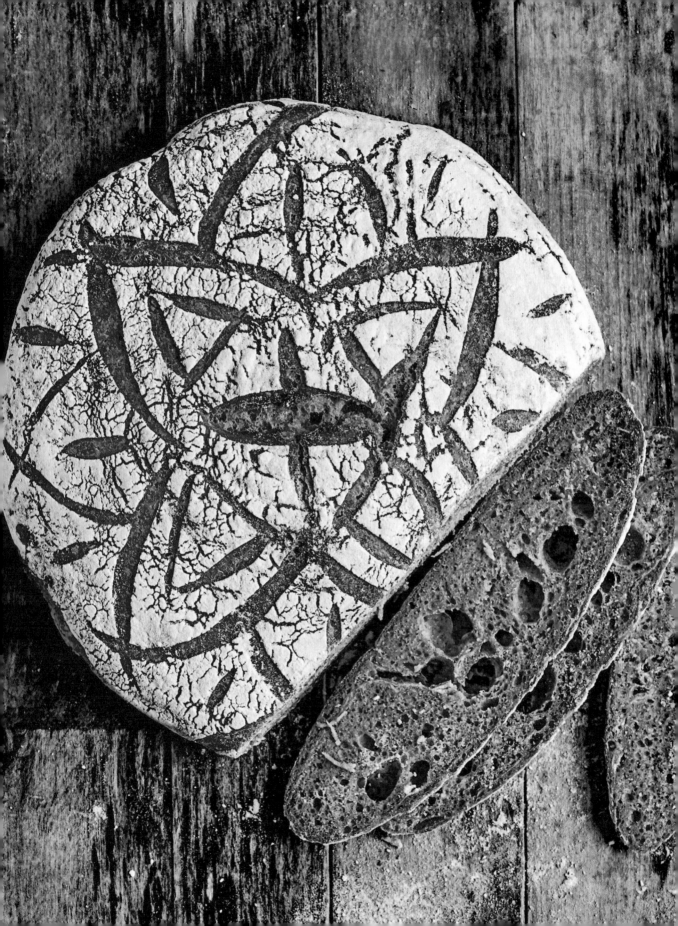

Flowerpot bread

Baking homemade bread is a chance for children to get involved in the kitchen, and flowerpots just add to the fun.

SERVES 5 · TAKES 50 mins plus rising

- 500g granary, strong, wholemeal or white bread flour
- 7g sachet fast-action dried yeast
- 2 tbsp olive oil, plus extra for the flowerpots
- 1 tbsp clear honey
- seeds, nuts, herbs or cheese, to top

1 Tip the flour, yeast and 1 tsp salt into a large bowl. Pour in 300ml warm water, the olive oil and honey. Mix with a wooden spoon until the mixture clumps together, then tip out onto a work surface. Use your hands to stretch and knead the dough for about 10 mins, or until it's smooth and springy. Add a little extra flour if the dough feels too sticky.

2 Brush the flowerpots with oil and line the sides with baking parchment. Divide the dough into 5 pieces and shape into smooth balls. Place 1 ball of dough into each flowerpot and cover with cling film. Leave in a warm place for 1 hr to rise.

3 Heat oven to 200C/180C fan/gas 6. When the dough has doubled in size, remove the cling film from the flowerpots and gently brush with a little oil. Sprinkle with your choice of topping.

4 Place the pots on a baking tray in the oven and cook for 20–25 mins until risen and golden. The pots will be very hot, so be careful when removing from the oven. Leave to cool for 10 mins before turning out and eating.

FLOWERPOTS
Clay flowerpots need to be treated to stop the bread from sticking. To do this, generously brush the pots with oil or butter and bake at 200C/180C fan/gas 5 for 1 hr. Remove from the oven, wash in hot soapy water, then dry before using.

Nutrition per loaf
Kcals 434 · fat 8g · saturates 1g · carbs 74g · sugars 4g · fibre 3g · protein 13g salt 1g

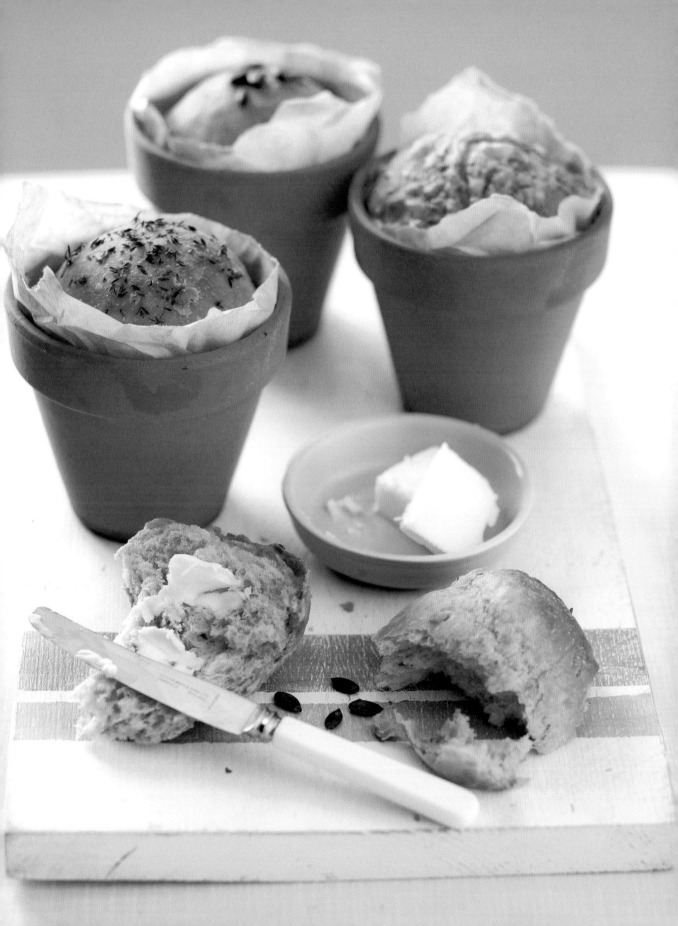

Triangular bread thins

Bake our easy bread thins with wholemeal spelt and top with your favourite ingredients for a healthy lunch.

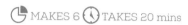 MAKES 6 ⏱ TAKES 20 mins

- 190g plain wholemeal spelt flour, plus extra for dusting
- ½ tsp bicarbonate of soda
- 1 tsp baking powder
- 75ml live bio yogurt made up to 150ml with cold water

1 Heat oven to 200C/180C fan/gas 6 and line a baking sheet with baking parchment. Mix the flour, bicarbonate of soda and baking powder in a bowl, then stir in the diluted yogurt with the blade of a knife until you have a soft, sticky dough, adding a little water if the mix is dry.

2 Tip the dough onto a lightly floured surface and shape and flatten with your hands to make a 20cm round. Take care not to over-handle as it can make the bread tough. Lift onto the baking sheet and cut into 6 triangles, slightly easing them apart with the knife. Bake for about 10–12 mins – they don't have to be golden, but should feel firm. Leave to cool on a wire rack. Pack into a food bag to use throughout the week, or freeze until needed.

Nutrition per triangle
Kcals 115 • fat 1g • saturates 0.3g • carbs 21g • sugars 1g • fibre 2g • protein 5g • salt 0.4g

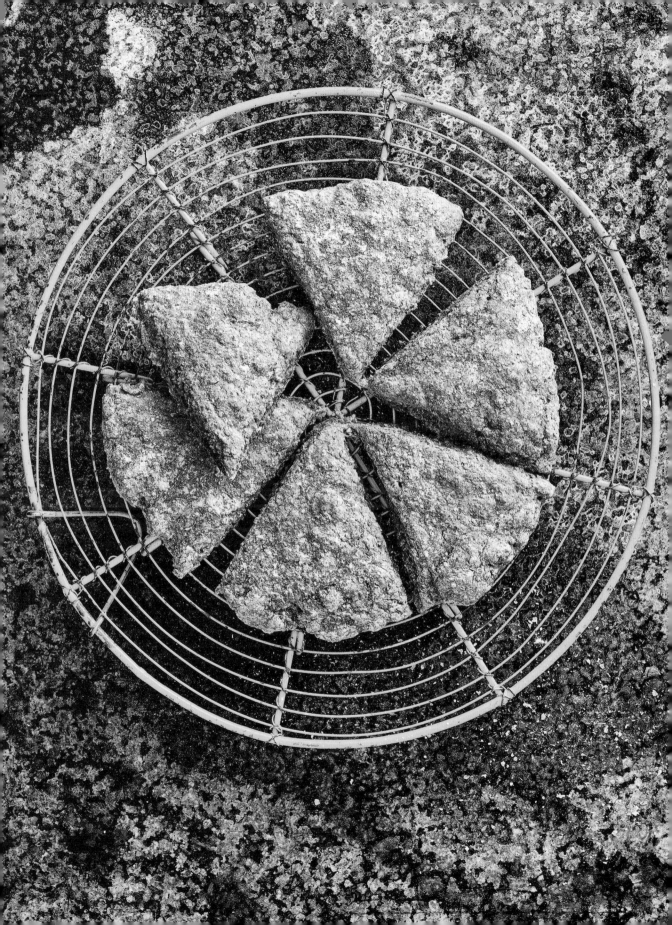

Chapatis

We can't resist a warm chapati with our favourite curry. This traditional Indian side dish is easier than you think and only takes a handful of ingredients.

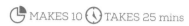 MAKES 10 TAKES 25 mins

- 140g wholemeal flour
- 140g plain flour, plus extra for dusting
- 1 tsp salt
- 2 tbsp olive oil, plus extra for greasing
- 180ml hot water or as needed

1 In a large bowl, stir together the flours and salt. Use a wooden spoon to stir in the olive oil and enough water to make a soft dough that is elastic but not sticky.

2 Knead the dough on a lightly floured surface for 5–10 mins until it is smooth. Divide into 10 pieces, or less if you want bigger breads. Roll each piece into a ball. Let rest for a few mins.

3 Heat a frying pan over medium heat until hot, and grease lightly. On a lightly floured surface, use a floured rolling pin to roll out the balls of dough until very thin like a tortilla.

4 When the pan starts smoking, put a chapati on it. Cook until the underside has brown spots, about 30 seconds, then flip and cook on the other side. Put on a plate and keep warm while you cook the rest of the chapatis.

Nutrition per serving
Kcals 121 • fat 3g • saturates 0.4g • carbs 20g • sugars 0.3g • fibre 2g • protein 3g • salt 0.5g

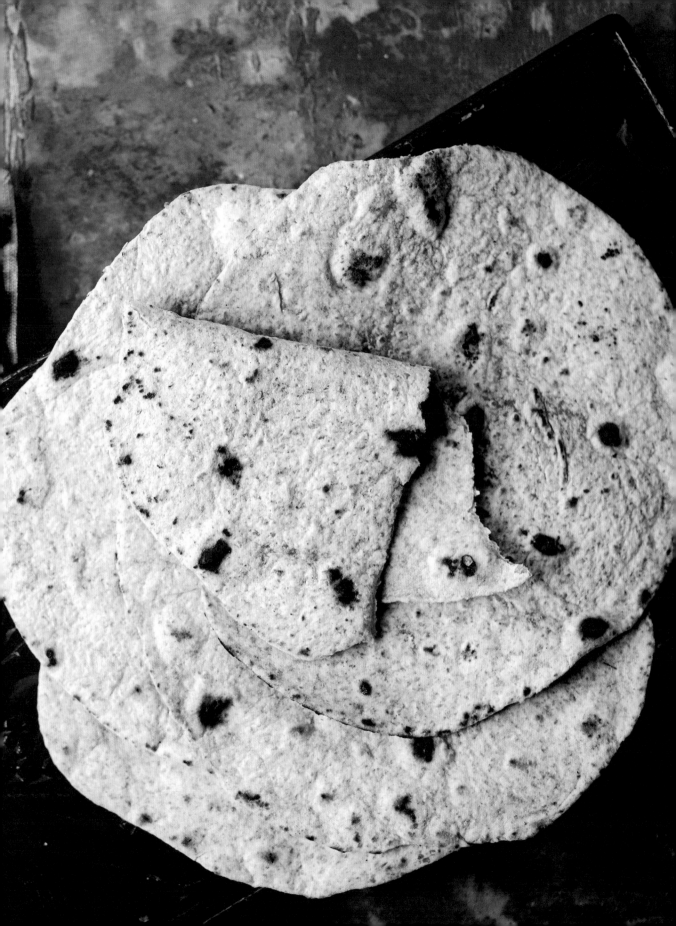

Index